Everything You Need To Know About Orthodontic Treatment:

An expert's guide with answers to frequently asked questions

Dr. J. Luke Chapman

EVERYTHING YOU NEED TO KNOW ABOUT
ORTHODONTIC TREATMENT: An Expert's Guide
With Answers To Frequently Asked Questions
by J. Luke Chapman, DDS

ISBN: 978-1496036100

Printed in the United States of America

First Edition

www.LukeChapmanOrtho.com

Table of Contents

Introduction

If you are thinking about starting orthodontic treatment to straighten your teeth or your child's teeth, you surely have a few questions. Maybe you have some concerns, fears, or anxiety. There is no doubt you are wondering how much this will hurt, and how much this will cost. You've heard horror stories from some of your friends about how much pain they experienced when they were kids and had braces. You've seen movies and television shows in which characters are unfortunate enough to have to wear some of these torture devices, such as a scary headgear or big metal wires. You may also have adult friends who are undergoing treatment right now, and you're wondering why they're doing it now and what kind of experience they are having. You're really wondering if this is going to hurt.

Here is some good news: orthodontics continues to change at a great pace. Huge advancements occur and make treatment both quicker and more comfortable for the patient. Each decade, newer advancements with products and techniques are made, enabling orthodontists to treat more complex cases with more beautiful results, which wouldn't have been possible a few years ago. Some techniques have been around for ages, and some are being tried and perfected with each ongoing year.

We get a lot of questions from our patients, both before starting their orthodontic treatment and during their treatment. The same questions seem to pop up, so you are not alone. This book is designed to answer most of those questions. You may not see a specific question listed in the Table of Contents main heading questions, but I'd bet the answer you're looking for is somewhere close in a related section.

I think for some patients the barrier to getting to the orthodontist's office or beginning treatment is really just being unsure about what to expect. I don't want these fears to prevent you or your child from getting the smile and the self-confidence you both deserve. Hopefully, this book will tell you just about everything you need to know before starting orthodontic treatment and help you overcome your concerns.

I want to let you know that no two orthodontists do things the same way. This book is a general guide on how things usually take place, like scheduling your first appointment and how braces and retainers work. Orthodontists vary greatly on the way appointments work in their office, the kinds of braces they use, the types of appliances and retainers they use, and the philosophies of treatment they practice. This book is intended to get your feet wet with what you should know about orthodontic treatment, and your orthodontist will fill you in on all the particulars that are suited to your specific needs and his specific treatment modalities.

All photographs of patients in this book, including before treatment, after treatment, during treatment, smiling photos, and profile photos are patients who were treated by the author in his private practice.

Part I

WHAT SHOULD I KNOW BEFORE BEGINNING ORTHODONTIC TREATMENT?

1

WHAT IS ORTHODONTICS?

Orthodontics is the specialty of dentistry that is focused on the diagnosis, prevention, and treatment of dental malocclusions, which may be a result of irregular tooth alignment (crowding or spacing), disproportionate jaw relationships, or both. Orthodontic treatment can be aimed at moving teeth to get them straighter, or it can be used to help control and modify facial growth. When orthodontic treatment tries to control the growth of jaws in growing children, it is called "dentofacial orthopedics."

The goals of orthodontic treatment include ideal dental (tooth) alignment and occlusion, ideal skeletal (jaw) relationships, with a comfortable, functional occlusion.

Simply put, orthodontic treatment tries to provide you with straight teeth in the proper place with facial and jaw balance, allowing you to chew and eat comfortably.

2

WHAT IS AN ORTHODONTIST?

Orthodontists are specialists who have completed an advanced education program beyond dental school to learn the special skills required to manage tooth movement and guide facial development. An additional 2-3 years are spent in an orthodontic residency after graduating from dental school. Orthodontists limit their practices to orthodontics; so fillings, dentures, and other areas of dentistry are eliminated. In an orthodontist's office, it is just orthodontics all the time.

The education of the orthodontist is never complete. He is required to complete continuing education throughout the entirety of his career. Look to see if he holds memberships in fundamental organizations such as the American Association of Orthodontists (AAO), the state component of the AOA, and the American Dental Association (ADA).

What is a board certified orthodontist?

An orthodontic specialist is eligible to become board certified through the *voluntary* examination process of the American Board of Orthodontics (ABO). Involvement in the certification process is a demonstration of the orthodontist's pursuit of continued proficiency and excellence. To become board certified, the orthodontist must complete a written examination demonstrating his knowledge on all aspects of orthodontics. After this, the orthodontist must present some of his treated cases in a clinical examination, where expert examiners and members of the Board evaluate the diagnosis and treatment performed by the candidate. Also, once certified, the orthodontist must re-examine on a periodic basis to maintain the board certified status. A board certified orthodontist earns the title of Diplomate of the ABO. It is worth mentioning that as of this writing, fewer than half of practicing orthodontists are certified by the American Board of Orthodontics.

No two orthodontists practice exactly the same way. Orthodontists use different kinds of braces and appliances. They schedule appointment times differently. Some choose shorter appointments scheduled closer together, and others will wait months before seeing you again, but keep you at the office a little longer during each visit. Some believe that to get the best treatment results for a certain malocclusion, you should extract some teeth, while other orthodontists will rarely if ever take out any teeth. Just keep in mind that no matter what the treatment philosophy of the orthodontist, the patient's best interest should be the center of his focus.

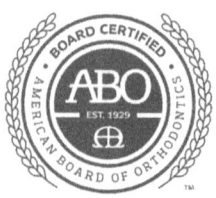

Figure 2-1. An example of the logo used by ABO certified orthodontists on letterhead and brochures.

3

THE BENEFITS OF ORTHODONTIC TREATMENT

Orthodontic treatment goals include providing ideal dental (tooth) alignment and bite, ideal skeletal (jaw) relationships, with a comfortable, functional occlusion. So, the orthodontist wants to provide straight teeth and a good bite. What does straight teeth do for you? There are physical and emotional benefits to straightening misaligned teeth.

The physical benefits of well-aligned teeth are the ones you can see. It is easy for others to notice your beautiful smile after orthodontic treatment. Your teeth will fit together better, allowing you better functioning during eating. Straight, well-aligned teeth are easier to floss and clean, leading to less gingivitis and better long-term health of the teeth and gums. Children with big front-to-back overbites (called overjet) and protrusive upper front teeth are more prone to traumatic injuries of those teeth. You are more likely to damage front teeth that stick out if you fall, play contact sports, or get hit with a basketball.

There are also emotional benefits gained when you undergo orthodontic treatment. Children know when their teeth are different than their friends' teeth.

Unfortunately, kids can be really ruthless in tormenting and teasing others with bucked teeth, crooked teeth, or large gaps. Correcting more severe problems like these can definitely reduce anxiety and self-consciousness in children during school age years. Both children and adults will have an increase in self-confidence when they can show off a big, full smile with well-aligned teeth. Whether it is a casual meeting or job interview, it is well known that one of the first things other people notice about you and create a first impression based on is your smile and teeth.

Orthodontics is not merely for improving the esthetics of the smile; orthodontic treatment improves bad bites (malocclusions). Malocclusions occur as a result of tooth or jaw misalignment. Malocclusions affect the way you smile, chew, clean your teeth, or feel about your smile.

So, a general list of benefits of orthodontic treatment follows:

- A more attractive smile
- Reduced appearance-consciousness during critical development years
- Better function of the teeth
- Possible increase in self-confidence
- Increased ability to clean the teeth
- Better long-term health of teeth and gums
- Guidance of permanent teeth into more favorable positions
- Reduction of the risk of injury to protruded front teeth
- Improved force distribution and wear patterns of the teeth
- Facilitation and enhancement of other dental treatment.

4

WHO COULD BENEFIT FROM ORTHODONTIC TREATMENT?

Orthodontic treatment can be successful at any age. Everyone wants a beautiful and healthy smile. Nearly anyone at any age can seek orthodontic treatment. You are never too old to get the smile you always wanted. In fact, more and more adults are seeking orthodontic treatment, and practices report up to 25% of their patients being older than 18. It may be beneficial for young children to postpone treatment until their early teenage years, but severe problems can be corrected as early as age 6, especially if social teasing is a concern.

Your dentist will point out specific problems to you and should let you know if you should see an orthodontist. Some problems are fairly visible, and you can recognize them in your child's mouth or your mouth.

Some of the most common orthodontic problems follow:

- Upper front teeth protrude excessively over the lower teeth, and are bucked
- Upper front teeth cover the majority of the lower teeth when biting together (deep bite)
- Upper front teeth are behind or inside the lower

front teeth (underbite) when biting together
- The upper and lower front teeth do not touch when biting together (open bite)
- Teeth are crowded or overlapped
- The center of the upper and lower teeth do not line up
- Finger or thumb sucking habits continue after six or seven years old
- Chewing is difficult
- Teeth are wearing unevenly or excessively
- The lower jaw shifts to one side when biting together
- Spaces are seen between the teeth.

Teeth have a specific way of fitting together when you bite. Top teeth are slightly outside of the bottom teeth in the back of your mouth. Top teeth are also slightly in front of your bottom teeth in the front of your mouth. There is supposed to be a little overlap of your front teeth, about 2 millimeters.

Anterior crossbites (Figure 4-1) happen when one or two of your top front teeth bite behind your bottom front teeth. The normal relationship of your front teeth "crosses over" when you bite. Besides looking unattractive, there are other concerns with this problem. This can result in abnormal wear of your front teeth, as the teeth are contacting in a way that they weren't designed to do. When enamel wears away, it doesn't grow back. If enough of the tooth structure is worn away, the teeth can become sensitive and be more prone to decay. Also, the way your teeth fit with a crossbite, the way they are supposed to fit, and the way your TMJ's (temperomandibular joints) want you to bite will not match and can lead to posturing your jaws forward in an abnormal way. Strong, abnormal forces are also placed on teeth with crossbites, which can lead to recession around those teeth (Figure 4-1). Anterior crossbites can be caused by permanent teeth erupting in the wrong direction or over-retention of baby teeth. These are usually corrected as early as possible.

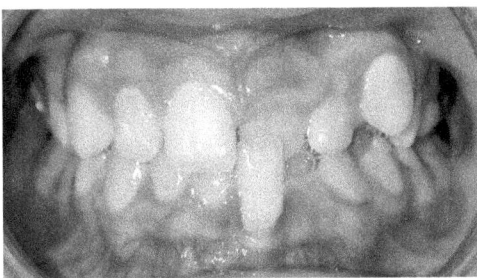

Figure 4-1. Anterior crossbite and recession on a lower incisor.

Posterior crossbites (Figures 4-2 and 4-3) happen when your top back teeth bite either too far inside your bottom teeth ("lingual crossbite") or too far on the outside of your bottom teeth ("buccal crossbite"). Posterior crossbites can be the result of permanent teeth erupting in the wrong directions, but these are most often the result of the top jaw being slightly small or narrow relative to the bottom jaw. So, there is a skeletal component to posterior crossbites, leading to more narrow maxillary arches. Similar consequences can result as with anterior crossbites. These can lead to abnormal wear on back teeth and other functional problems. Also, these usually lead to an abnormal shifting of the jaw to one side when you function and is noticed when the dental midlines don't line up (Figure 4-4). The way the teeth actually fit and the way your TMJ's want them to fit aren't in harmony, which can lead to breakdown of the teeth, periodontal structures, or the TMJ's. These are usually corrected as early as possible.

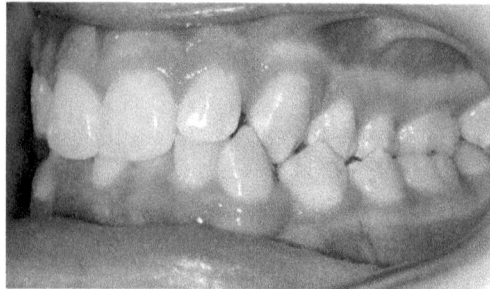

Figure 4-2. Posterior crossbite.

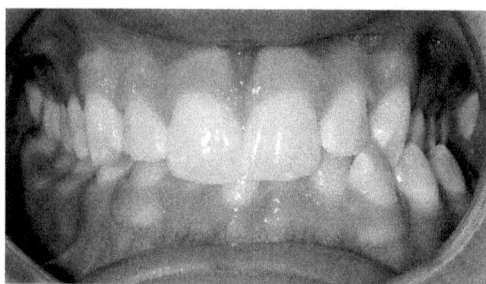

Figure 4-3. Posterior crossbite (same patient as Figure 2).

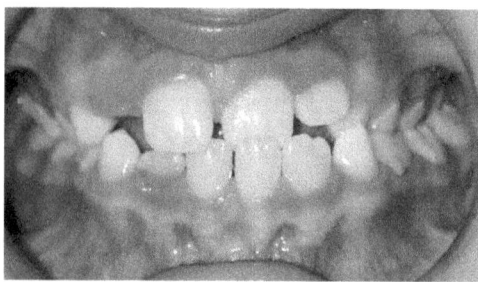

Figure 4-4. Posterior and anterior crossbites with midline and jaw shifting to the side.

Crowding (Figure 4-5) is a dental irregularity where teeth look crooked. Teeth are misaligned and look out of place. This may be a result of the permanent teeth not erupting in the correct position, keeping baby teeth too long, having large teeth, having small jaws, or not having enough room in the jaw to accommodate all the teeth. Crowding can happen with top or bottom teeth. Crowding is both an esthetic problem and a functional problem. Crooked teeth don't look pretty in a smile and can lead to self-consciousness, causing you to hold back

smiles in social interactions. Crooked and rotated teeth
are hard to properly clean and can lead to plaque buildup.
Teeth that are severely out of place may fit with the
opposing teeth in an abnormal way and lead to abnormal
wearing way of enamel. Sometimes, crowding is so
severe that permanent teeth will have to be taken out to
make room for the rest of the teeth present. This usually
isn't an emergency to treat, and your orthodontist will
recommend the best time to treat and the best course of
action to take for your child. Adults can usually fix this
any time he or she desires.

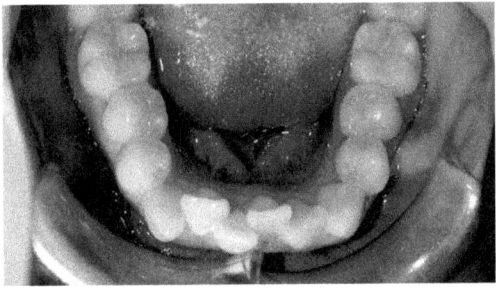

*Figure 4-5.
Crowding of
bottom teeth.*

Overbites come in two varieties. "Overbite" is the
dental term that refers to the vertical (top to bottom)
overlap of the front teeth. A typical overbite is about 2
millimeters. "Overjet" is the dental term that refers to
the horizontal (front to back) distance between the top
front teeth and the bottom front teeth. A typical overjet
is about 2 millimeters. Most patients will say, "I have an
overbite," but they are referring to their overjet. Overjet
problems are usually more noticeable and worrisome for
patients seeking treatment; overbite problems are only
noticed when patients bite down fully.

A **deep bite** (Figure 4-6) happens when there is too
much vertical (up-down) overlap of the front teeth when
the patient bites. Extra force is placed upon the lower
front teeth. This leads to abnormal and accelerated wear
of these incisors. Often, the lower front teeth wear down
and an alarming rate. Also, the extra force can lead to

recession around these teeth. This can be a problem that is caused by the teeth alone, or sometimes the direction of growth of the jaws can lead to a deep bite. This problem is sometimes treated as early as possible, depending on how fast the teeth are wearing down, how much the skeletal component contributes to the problem, where the child is in development, and what the orthodontist's philosophy dictates.

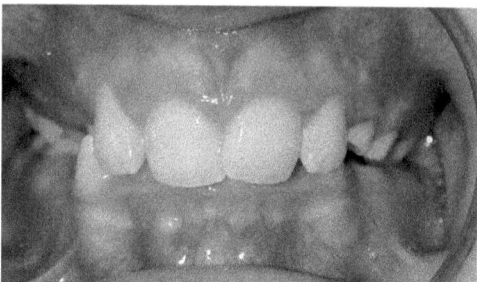

Figure 4-6.
Deep bite.

Excess **overjet** (Figure 4-7) occurs when the horizontal (front to back) distance between the top front teeth and bottom front teeth is too large. The maxillary incisors are said to be "bucked" teeth, are too protrusive, and stick out too far. A finger-sucking habit can lead to protrusive incisors. Often, there is a jaw growth problem, where the lower jaw is set back relative to the top jaw. The lower jaw is too small and is described as mandibular retrognathism. This is an obviously unsightly problem to have, and it is a frequent cause of schoolyard picking and teasing. Also, maxillary incisors that are protrusive are more likely to experience a traumatic emergency. A blow to the face during contact sports, ball games, or even a fall is more likely to result in damage to these front teeth. The teeth can chip, crack, loosen, or totally avulse (get knocked out). This bite is usually part of what orthodontists call a Class II malocclusion. Class II refers to a bite where the lower teeth all bite behind where they are supposed to fit with the upper teeth. If the lower jaw is small and set too far back, then all the teeth will fit too far back also. Excess overjet is usually corrected as early as it is discovered. The orthodontist may begin growth modification techniques to address the skeletal growth problems at an early age, maybe around age 9.

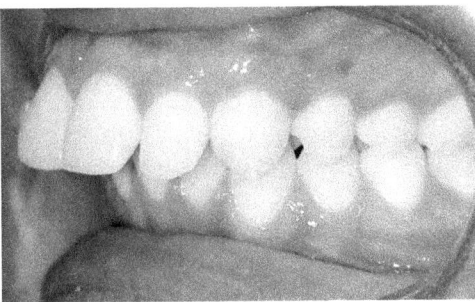

Figure 4-7.
Excess overjet.

Anterior open bites (Figure 4-8) happen when the patient bites down and there is no vertical overlap of the top and bottom front teeth. There can be a gap between the maxillary and mandibular incisors when the patient bites, and the patient's tongue may be visible. These can result from a finger-sucking habit, a tongue posture habit, or a vertical growth discrepancy between the two jaws. Open bites can cause speech problems, as the tongue cannot properly form sounds against the teeth. Sometimes there is extra wear on the back teeth because they bear all of the forces of functioning. Open bites with speech difficulty are addressed as early as possible so that the child can begin proper functioning and speech patterns (sometimes with the help of a speech therapist). Finger-habits after the age of 6 are cause for concern and usually addressed at this time. Mild open bites or open bites discovered later may be treated at a later time, if the orthodontist would prefer to allow all permanent teeth to erupt or allow for more growth.

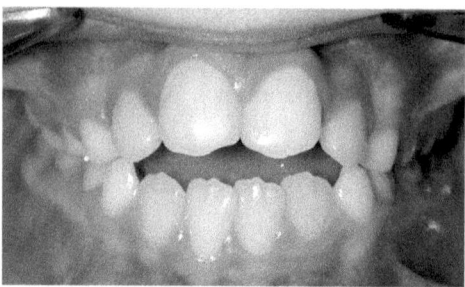

Figure 4-8. Anterior open bite.

Posterior or **lateral open bites** (Figure 4-9) occur when the back teeth don't touch as the patient bites. There is a vertical space between the top and bottom back teeth on one side or both sides. These can result from permanent teeth that fail to come in all the way, from ankylosed teeth, from a tongue posturing habit, or from jaw growth discrepancies. Lateral open bites can cause asymmetric jaw shifting and difficulty with functioning. Also, the teeth that do touch may wear down as the forces of mastication are spread unevenly. These are usually treated around age 12 or later if they are discovered at a later time.

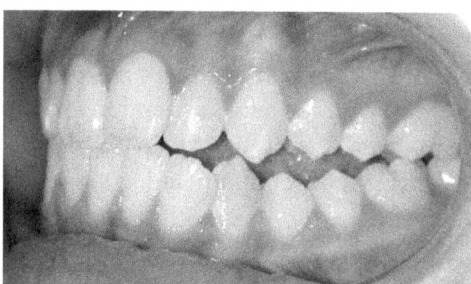

Figure 4-9. Lateral or posterior open bite.

Spacing (Figure 4-10) is seen as gaps between teeth in the same arch. The teeth do not touch their neighbors. Reasons for excess spacing include smaller than average teeth, large jaws, jaw growth problems, unerupted permanent teeth, impacted teeth, and congenitally missing teeth. Excess gaps are unattractive in a smile. Sometimes other procedures will be indicated to fully correct spacing problems, like surgeries to expose and orthodontically erupt impacted and ectopic teeth, and restorative procedures to bond build-ups to small teeth. Most spacing problems can be treated in the age 12 to 13 time frame after enough time is given for unerupted teeth to spontaneously erupt on their own.

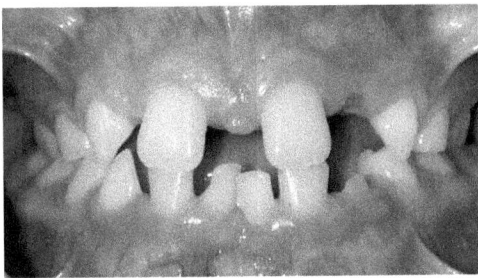

Figure 4-10.
Excess spacing.

Underbites (Figure 4-11) happen when most of the top front teeth are behind some bottom front teeth when the patient bites. True underbites are indicative of skeletal growth problems where the mandible is growing too far forward relative of the maxilla. Some underbites are mild and result in the patient posturing the lower jaw forward to have the teeth come together more comfortably. Underbites can lead to abnormal wear on some the teeth, TMJ concerns if the lower jaw is habitually postured forward, and permanent skeletal disharmonies. Underbites can be part of what orthodontists call a Class III malocclusion. Class III bites are when the lower jaw grows farther forward compared to the upper jaw. As the lower jaw goes forward, the lower teeth follow and are in front of the top teeth. Similarly, if the maxilla doesn't grow enough, Class III bites can result. Underbites are usually treated as early as possible.

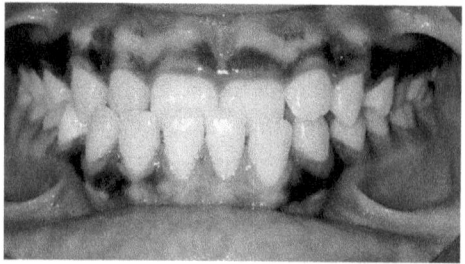

Figure 4-11.
Underbite.

Buccal corridors (Figure 4-12) are the dark spaces between the cheeks and the teeth in a person's smile. There can be extra space or dark shadows around the corners of the mouth and the back teeth. Narrow maxillary arches or misaligned teeth can cause them. It is generally considered more esthetically pleasing to have a broader, fuller smile that fills in the spaces next to your lips when you smile. Compare the smiles before and after orthodontic treatment in the two adults in Figures 4-12 through 4-15 and one teenager (Figure 4-16 and 4-17).

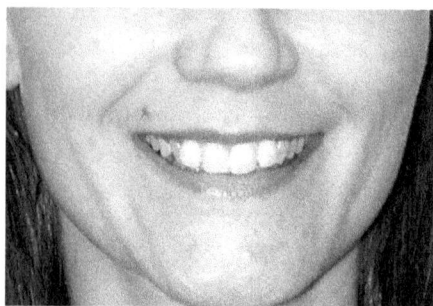

Figure 4-12. Buccal corridors and shadows with a narrow arch before orthodontic treatment.

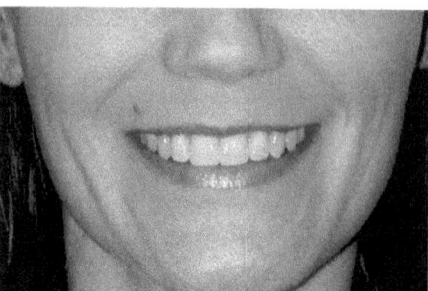

Figure 4-13. Broad smile and eliminated buccal corridors after orthodontic treatment (patient from Figure 4-12.)

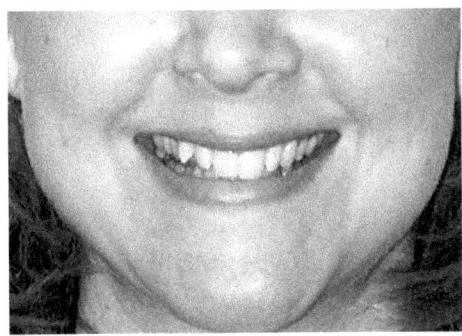

Figure 4-14. Narrow arches and smile with buccal corridors before orthodontic treatment.

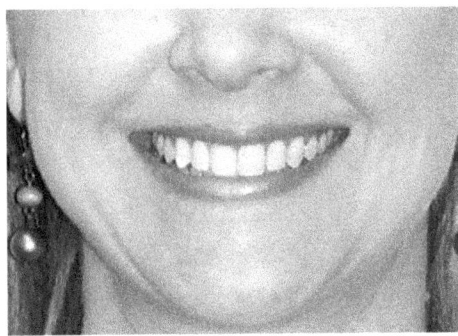

Figure 4-15. Broader and improved smile after orthodontic treatment (patient from Figure 4-14).

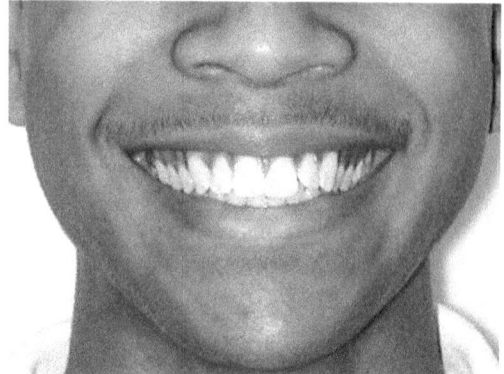

Figure 4-16. Smile with buccal corridors and upper teeth that lean towards the tongue.

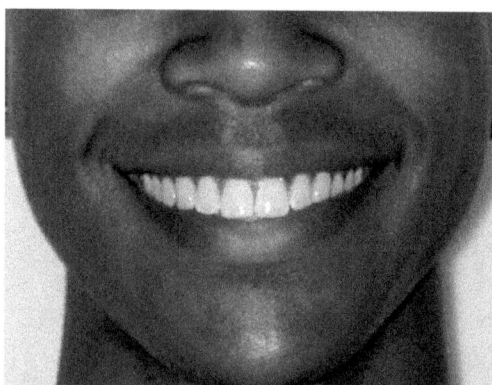

Figure 4-17. Broader and improved smile with upright upper teeth after treatment (patient from Figure 4-16).

The above examples are just a few of the most common orthodontic problems that can occur. Others not shown here are less obvious to parents and patients. Your dentist may have to point them out, and he may only be able to see these problems on an x-ray. Some other examples include impacted teeth, ectopically erupting teeth, transposed teeth, ankylosed teeth, supernumerary (extra) teeth, or congenitally missing teeth.

Skeletal Problems

When the maxilla and the mandible grow disproportionately to one another, skeletal malocclusions result. The fit of the teeth is severely off, and a bad malocclusion will exist. Jaw disharmonies can be seen in the patient's face; it may look like a deficient chin or a protruding lower jaw. These skeletal malocclusions should be addressed as soon as possible. If an orthodontist sees a child at age 7, growth modification can begin early while the child is growing. Modification of jaw growth after the age of 12 or 13 is unlikely, as beneficial growth spurts are complete at this age. If skeletal disharmonies are bad enough, an orthognathic surgery to fix the jaws may be the only way to get the teeth to fit properly.

A Class I jaw relationship occurs when there is proportionate, correct growth of the upper and lower jaws. The face will look well balanced. The forehead, upper lip, and chin will nearly line up in profile (Figure 4-18).

Class II jaw relationships happen when the lower jaw is small or set back relative to the upper jaw. The chin will look small or deficient, and the lower third of the face usually looks short (Figure 4-19).

Class III jaw relationships happen when the upper jaw is small or set back relative to the lower jaw. The chin will look like it is too far in front of the face. The patient looks like he has an underbite (Figure 4-20).

Figure 4-18.   Class I profiles.

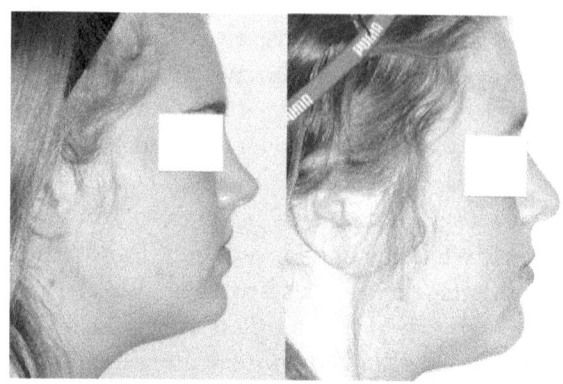

Figure 4-19.   Class II profiles.

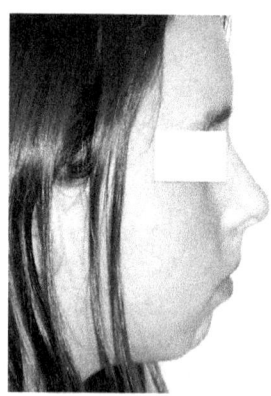 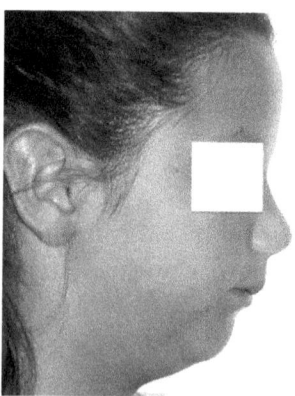

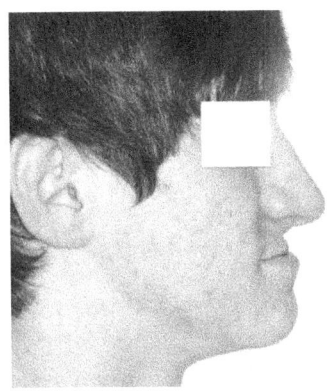

Figure 4-20. Class III profile.

Why should malocclusions be treated?

According to studies by the American Association of Orthodontists, untreated malocclusions can result in a variety of problems. Crowded teeth are more difficult to properly brush and floss, which may contribute to tooth decay and/or gum disease. Protruding teeth are more susceptible to accidental chipping and traumatic injuries. Crossbites can result in unfavorable growth and uneven tooth wear. Open bites can result in tongue-thrusting habits and speech impediments. Over-crowding can lead to "blocked out" teeth, or teeth that don't have enough space to erupt. If these teeth don't erupt, they can become impacted and stuck in the jaw bone. Impacted teeth can cause damage to the roots of the adjacent teeth or cause pain and inflammation. Ultimately, orthodontics does more than make a pretty smile—it creates a healthier, happier, more confident you.

5

WHY DID MY DENTIST RECOMMEND ORTHODONTIC TREATMENT?

During a routine visit to your general dentist, he may say that you or your child is "ready to see an orthodontist." If your dentist is recommending an orthodontic consultation, he sees one or more of the above problems, either in a mild form or a more severe form. The general dentist's job is to make you aware of the problem that he sees and refer you to the orthodontic specialist. Although the dentist is recommending that you see an orthodontist now, your orthodontist may decide that you are not ready for treatment now. The orthodontic specialist will discuss your orthodontic problems, explain how these problems are fixed, and specify when these problems should be treated.

Do I need a referral from a dentist to see an orthodontist?

No, you don't need a referral from a dentist to see an orthodontist. You are welcome to call and schedule an exam with an orthodontist if you want to discuss you or your child's teeth and treatment options even without a direct referral or recommendation from your general dentist. If the orthodontist needs more diagnostic information, like current x-rays, which your dentist may have, then the orthodontist may request copies before your appointment or after you have met.

6

TREATMENT FOR CHILDREN

The American Association of Orthodontists recommends that all children be evaluated by an orthodontist at the age of 7. That does sound young! By the age of 7, the first adult molars erupt, establishing the bite, and the adult incisors also erupt. During this time, an orthodontist can evaluate front-to-back and side-to-side tooth relationships. For example, the presence of erupting incisors can indicate possible overbite, open bite, crowding, or gummy smiles. Timely screening increases the chances for an incredible smile. However, at this age serious skeletal growth patterns can be discerned, and appropriate treatment can be planned.

It's best for the orthodontist to see children by age 7 to advise if orthodontic treatment is required, and if it is the best time for that patient to be treated. Any crossbites, crowding, and other problems can be evaluated at that time. At this early age, orthodontic treatment may not be necessary, but vigilant examination can anticipate the most advantageous time to begin treatment. There are many advantages of waiting to initiate treatment until the adolescent years, and most often treatment is started in the teenage years. However, treatment in the early preteen years can be beneficial in certain individuals.

Timing is everything with orthodontic treatment. Treatment aimed at guiding the jaws to grow to a better position or relationship should be started well before all of the permanent teeth are erupted and while the child is actively growing. Some psychosocial benefits can be gained in treating severely misaligned teeth on a limited basis while there are still baby teeth present, especially if the child is being teased in school. *The vast majority of 7-year-olds will not need orthodontic treatment.* The gold standard of timing orthodontic treatment is beginning at age 12 or 13 with most kids, as this is the age that all permanent teeth are erupted or close to being seen in the mouth. So, age 7 is important, and it is never too early to have a plan.

When treatment begins early, the orthodontist can guide the growth of the jaws and guide incoming permanent teeth. Early treatment can also regulate the width of the upper and lower dental arches, gain space for permanent teeth, help to avoid the need for permanent tooth extractions, reduce the likelihood of impacted permanent teeth, correct thumb-sucking, and eliminate abnormal swallowing or speech problems. In other words, when indicated early treatment can simplify later treatment.

So, orthodontic treatment can be started at any age. Many orthodontic problems are easier to correct if detected at an early age before jaw growth has slowed. Early treatment may mean that a patient can avoid surgery and more serious complications. Beginning treatment at this time ensures the greatest result and the least amount of time and expense. For some, it would be an advantage to start early treatment in the preteen years, but most often, it is best to start during adolescence.

The following is a summary of the results of early, interceptive treatment in children:

- Create room for crowded, erupting teeth
- Create facial symmetry by influencing jaw growth

- Reduce the risk of trauma to protruding front teeth
- Preserve space for unerupted teeth
- Reduce the need for permanent tooth removal
- Reduce total treatment time with full braces.

7

TREATMENT FOR ADULTS

Braces aren't just for kids anymore. Teeth can be straightened at any age if your gums and bone structure are healthy. Orthodontists offer a variety of treatments that are designed for different age groups, especially adults. Esthetic clear brackets or clear aligners can be used for many patients, virtually eliminating the appearance of wearing braces. It's never too late to improve your greatest asset, your smile.

Orthodontic treatment at later stages in life can dramatically improve your personal appearance and self-esteem. Improving the health of your teeth and gums is equally important. Crooked teeth and a bad bite can contribute to gum disease and bone loss, tooth decay, abnormal wear of the tooth enamel surfaces, headaches and jaw joint (TMJ/TMD) pain.

Here is some good news. New techniques and appliances have come around that greatly reduce discomfort levels, decrease the frequency of visits, and shorten treatment time. During the initial examination, your orthodontist will determine the best possible treatment for your individual needs. During this initial examination, he will outline the treatment plan, time of treatment expected, and the approximate cost.

Occasionally, jaw surgery is required for adult orthodontic patients because their jaw discrepancies need to be corrected in order to correct the patient's bite. Adults also may have already experienced some breakdown or loss of their teeth and bone that supports the teeth and may require periodontal treatment before, during, and/or after orthodontic treatment. Bone loss can also limit the amount and direction of tooth movement that is advisable.

The American Association of Orthodontists conducted a survey to ask adults about the improvements they had in their lives after completing orthodontic treatment with an orthodontist. The results were outstanding:

> 83% reported improved personal relationships.

> 58% reported improved career success.

> 92% of treated adults would recommend orthodontic treatment to other adults.

Positive outcomes included more confidence in the workplace and less stress and fear of judgment because they felt more self-assured when they smiled fully with straight teeth.

You can live the rest of your life with a beautiful smile if you choose to.

8

WHAT WILL HAPPEN DURING MY FIRST VISIT TO THE ORTHODONTIST'S OFFICE?

At your initial appointment, you will get to meet some of the key staff members and the orthodontist. The orthodontist will complete a thorough examination and discuss your orthodontic problems or malocclusion. He will also present potential treatment options and the possible benefits and consequences of each option. Also, he will inform you of the best time to start treatment and how long treatment will last. You will also get an idea of how much the treatment should cost. This examination appointment is usually short.

Some orthodontists may choose to take one or multiple radiographs (x-rays) or photographs at this visit to better diagnose and discuss your orthodontic needs. Otherwise, the x-rays will be made at the following visit.

During the initial examination, the following questions will be addressed: Is treatment needed now, or should treatment be delayed until appropriate growth, tooth eruption, or other factors have occurred? What treatment procedures will be used to correct my problems, or how will we fix this? Do any baby teeth or permanent teeth need to be removed? How long will treatment take? How much will it cost? What are my payment options?

While these general questions about treatment can be answered during the initial examination, the orthodontist will confirm his diagnosis and treatment plan details after careful analysis of diagnostic records. These records may be made at the initial visit or a subsequent visit depending on your available time or the orthodontist's preference.

How long does orthodontic treatment take? Treatment times vary on a case-by-case basis, but the average time is from one to two years. The rate of jaw growth, severity of the problem, and difficulty of the necessary correction can affect actual treatment time. More severe cases take longer than milder cases. Treatment length is also dependent upon patient compliance. Following instructions, maintaining good oral hygiene, and keeping regular appointments are important factors for keeping treatment time on schedule.

9

WHAT ARE ORTHODONTIC DIAGNOSTIC RECORDS?

Diagnostic records are essential pieces of information gathered by the orthodontist prior to beginning any orthodontic treatment. The records include orthodontic x-rays, photos, bite records, and impressions for study models of your teeth, and any other diagnostic information your orthodontist sees as beneficial to your treatment. The records are necessary for developing the appropriate treatment plan for you and to disclose any pertinent information about the health of your teeth, gums, and jaws. This additional appointment lasts approximately 30 minutes to one hour. It is necessary for the orthodontist to analyze each patient's specific and individual needs because in-depth planning leads to superior results and higher patient satisfaction.

What are impressions? Impressions may be a new experience for you and especially younger patients. Traditionally, a thick putty-like material that resembles bread dough is placed in a tray that fits in your mouth. The tray and putty are pressed against your teeth and flows to cover all of your teeth and gums. After about 30 seconds to a minute, the putty becomes more rigid and the tray is removed. Now the orthodontist has an impression or mold of your teeth (Figure 9-1). It is analogous to a bear's footprint left behind in soft mud. Next, a material that resembles plaster of Paris is mixed and poured into the impression. Once the plaster sets up and becomes solid, the orthodontist pulls the stone model out of the impression, and the orthodontist has a stone model of your teeth to study. He will do certain measurements with the stone model to give more information about your diagnosis. He may even attach the models of your teeth to a tool called an articulator (Figure 9-2). This allows your bite or occlusion to be clearly studied, as you can see how your top and bottom teeth really come together.

Technology continues to change the impression experience. More orthodontists are using digital impression scanning technology, which allows the orthodontist to forget about that putty. A special camera is placed in your mouth, a series of digital images are made, and digital models are created on a computer. Also, digital models can be made to plastic hand-held models with a 3-D printer.

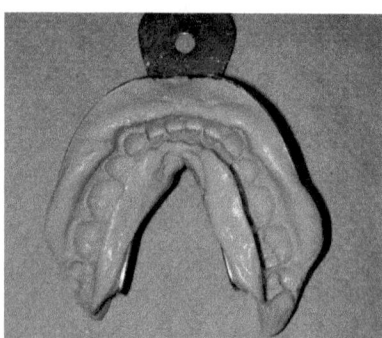

Figure 9-1. An impression of teeth.

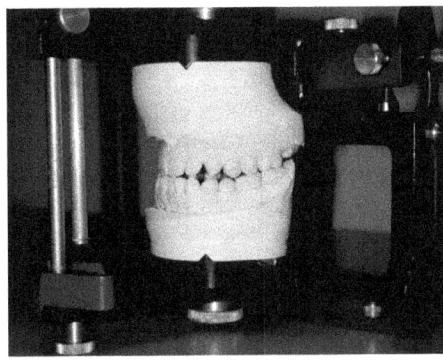

Figure 9-2.
Stone models of
teeth mounted on
an articulator.

The orthodontist may take x-rays to measure and assess the relationships of the jaws and the health of the teeth. 3-D scans of the head and jaws may be indicated. As technology improves, 3-D scans provide a dynamic range of diagnostic information, including accurate visualization of impacted teeth and even detailed measurements of airway volumes.

Next, the treatment coordinator will schedule a consultation visit to discuss your treatment options, time frames, and financial arrangements. This series of initial appointments will ultimately leave you with a clear understanding of your specific needs, the type of treatment you will receive, and how long it will take. Also, any other questions you may have can be answered all before your treatment begins. This ensures that you and the orthodontist are on the same page, so to speak, and helps to avoid any surprises later.

At this point, you will be ready to schedule your appointments to begin treatment and finalize your financial plans. Occasionally, additional information may be needed from your dentist or another dental specialist to better assess your overall dental treatment (like future restorative implants or periodontal concerns). A separate consultation with that doctor could be beneficial to further explore your treatment options and prognosis.

Some orthodontists will modify the number of visits it takes to initially examine you, complete the diagnostic records, and review the records and treatment plan with you. In some offices the initial examination, diagnostic records, treatment discussion/conference, and even the placement of braces can be done in one or two appointments. The important thing is to make sure you feel comfortable with the treatment expectations, comfortable with the office staff and policies, and comfortable with the treating orthodontist before your treatment begins.

10

HOW MUCH DOES TREATMENT COST?

The cost of orthodontic treatment varies greatly depending on the type of treatment used, the timing of treatment, the complexity of treatment, the type and number of appliances used, the orthodontist, and other regional and multifactorial differences. Quotes over the phone will give you an estimate of an average treatment, but the only way to get an accurate cost of treatment is for you to be examined by the orthodontist. It should be noted that differences in prices between orthodontists might reflect differences in treatment modalities and treatment goals. It is important to compare "apples to apples," as one orthodontist may be quoting more comprehensive care than the more inexpensive doctor. Also, the inexpensive doctor may not be quoting the cost of retainers or other treatment aspects upfront, and these costs may be presented later in treatment.

So, the only way to get an accurate cost of your treatment or your child's treatment is to actually go to the orthodontist's office. Remember that what your neighbor may have paid for his treatment probably won't be the same as what your treatment will cost…even with the same orthodontist! Don't think that what he was quoted for his treatment will necessarily be the same for you or your child.

There are different ways for patients to pay for treatment. Of course, checks and cash are usually welcome. Most offices take credit cards and debit cards too. Automatic bank drafts are sometimes available. You may have dental insurance with orthodontic benefits. This is great, as your out of pocket personal costs would be reduced! Be aware that not all dental insurance plans have orthodontic coverage. The orthodontic benefits vary dramatically among insurance carriers and plans. It is important to specifically inquire about "orthodontic" coverage when you establish a dental insurance plan. Insurance coverage can range from $500 $2500. Note also that there are age restrictions for some plans. Some plans provide "lifetime" coverage with no age limit. Also, the landscape of insurance policies and coverage is a fluid landscape that is always changing. Most offices will be happy to get your insurance information and contact the carriers to determine your benefits, and most offices will file the claims for you when treatment begins. Some other benefits and arrangements from your employment may come in handy. Flex plans are sometimes available and allow you to use these benefits on a time specific basis.

To learn more about your options, ask the office staff at your initial visit or when you are on the phone scheduling the initial visit. Most offices will be happy to assist you and maximize the benefits that are available to you. Clearly provide all information on the financial/insurance forms that the office provides to you. This will expedite process of determining your insurance coverage.

Most offices will not require you to pay the entire fee upfront. It is customary for orthodontic offices to collect a down payment before treatment begins. This will usually vary from 5% to 50% of the treatment cost. The remainder of the balance is usually financed. Many offices offer in-house financing with little or no interest charges over the length of the treatment duration.

Payments are usually made on a monthly basis. Sometimes, third party financers are necessary and are available at competitive interest rates, depending on your credit score.

Part II

WHAT SHOULD I EXPECT DURING ORTHODONTIC TREATMENT?

11

WHAT ARE BRACES?

Orthodontic braces or brackets are the tiny appliances that orthodontists cement or temporarily glue to your teeth. There are different kinds and shapes with different prescriptions built into them. The most common braces are the ones you see when people smile. They are bonded to the front or facial surfaces of the teeth. Built into the bracket is a slot where an orthodontic archwire fits. There are different sizes and shapes of archwires, and they are made of different metal alloys. The archwire is held in the braces by a ligature. Elastomeric O-shaped ligatures come in a variety of colors and should be changed on a regular basis. There are also steel ligatures, which are smaller and hold less plaque. Some braces are self-ligating and can hold the wire with built-in mechanisms, such as clips or doors, which eliminates the need for elastomeric ligature O-rings.

The brackets are simply a means of holding the archwire. The archwires do all the work of moving the teeth. Early in treatment small, super elastic, and super flexible archwires are used with light forces. As you progress through treatment, stronger, more resilient wires are used to fully engage the bracket and move the teeth to the final optimal positions. Orthodontists make adjustments to your braces by changing to a new shape of wire or a different material. Also, he can add bends to the archwire to move teeth.

Braces use steady gentle pressure to gradually move teeth into their proper positions. The initial archwire is placed in the brackets and may look like it makes zig zags and funny bends. Slowly and gently, the archwire tries to return to its original shape. As it does so, it applies pressure to move your teeth to their new, more ideal positions.

12

THE DIFFERENT KINDS OF BRACES

There are different types of braces. They can be placed on different areas of your teeth. Brackets can come in various shapes and sizes. Some are clear and barely noticeable. Some appliances act like braces but aren't braces at all.

The most commonly seen and used braces are bonded to the front of your teeth, next to your cheeks and lips. Orthodontists call that surface of your teeth the buccal, labial, or facial surface. These brackets are easily manipulated and accurately placed on the teeth because the orthodontist can easily see and visualize the facial surfaces of teeth. These brackets really show when you smile, and that is why kids get excited about having colors on their braces. They can flash their favorite colors every time they smile. Braces on the front of people's teeth are what you probably visualize when you think about orthodontic treatment. These are the most versatile and can be used to treat any type of malocclusion.

Metal braces

Traditionally, metal braces (Figure 12-1) have been the standard of orthodontic treatment. Their strength and durability make them very effective and desirable for orthodontic therapy. The colored "O" elastics (Figure 12-2) are made for metal brackets. The colors are not just for customizing the look of your braces. The colored "O's" are tiny rubber bands that hold the archwire inside the bracket. The elastic "O's" fade and accumulate plaque over time, so they must be changed on a regular basis. There are also elastic chains that are basically a string of "O's" connected together in a line. Chains are used to ligate the brackets and to close spaces. Metal ligatures can take the place of the elastic "O's" and are considered to be more hygienic and less plaque catching.

Other brackets eliminate the need for the plaque-collecting elastic "O's." These brackets are called self-ligating brackets because they hold the archwire with built in mechanisms, such as doors or clips (Figure 12-3). Self-ligating braces provide many advantages to the older braces with colored ties. The new self-ligating brackets offer smaller, more hygienic appliances that are easier to clean. Smaller, more narrow brackets provide more gentle forces to the teeth. Adjustment appointments are quicker because self-ligating braces are very easy to open and change wires; changing the elastic "O's" takes longer to tie the archwire in the brackets.

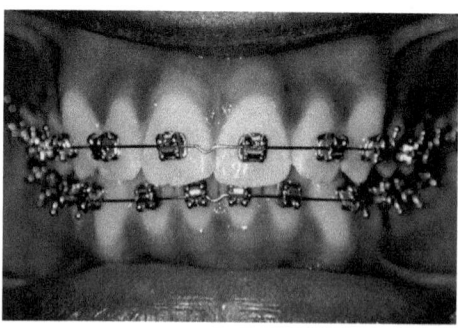

Figure 12-1. Metal self-ligating brackets.

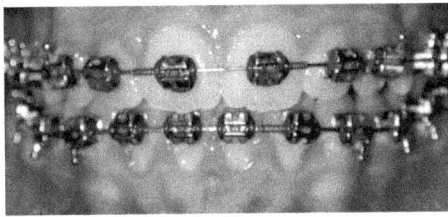

*Figure 12-2.
Colored elastic
"O's" around
metal braces.*

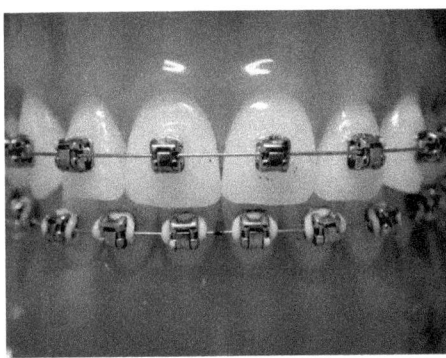

*Figure 12-3.
Metal self-ligating
brackets with and
without elastic "O"
colors.*

Ceramic tooth-colored braces

Ok, not everyone wants to show a mouth full of metal when they smile, and bright colors aren't a good option for them either. There is an answer. Ceramic tooth-colored braces are a great option for patients who really don't want metal braces and who want their braces to show very little. These are usually referred to as "clear" braces. The new self-ligating ceramic brackets offer superior esthetics as they look great and blend in with the natural teeth, and appointments are shorter and quicker because of the easy-to-open self-ligating technology. Other tooth-colored brackets can be made of special plastics. Ceramic brackets do not stain or change colors. The "O" rings traditionally used on ceramic brackets are clear. These clear elastics do absorb different pigments from your diet (coffee, soft drinks, ketchup) and stain fairly quickly. More frequent visits to change the dirty

"O's" may be needed. However, newer ceramic self-ligating brackets don't need the "O's," and there is no staining at all.

Are there any differences between metal and ceramic braces? Generally, both work on the same principles, and one is not faster than the other. Neither provides you with a shorter time in braces. Ceramic brackets are basically made of a strong glass. To withstand the forces of chewing, the ceramic is a little thicker to provide extra strength and prevent fracturing. So, some ceramic brackets are a little bigger than the metal counterparts. Bigger brackets can trap extra plaque, as they are harder and bulkier to clean, and bigger brackets stick out more, leading to a greater chance of being in the way when you bite. Some orthodontists will bond the smaller, metal brackets on the lower teeth to avoid your biting on them. Also, some orthodontists choose not to use clear brackets, and some charge extra to use them. Figure 12-4 shows ceramic brackets, and Figure 12-5 shows the brackets with elastic chain.

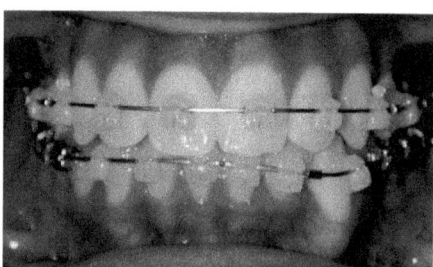

Figure 12-4.
Ceramic self-ligated
brackets.

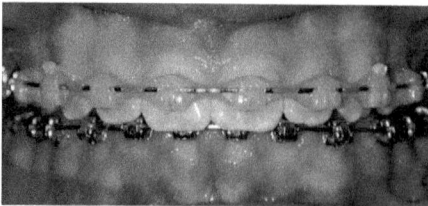

Figure 12-5.
Elastic chain
around clear
brackets .

Braces enhanced by digital technology

New technology allows the orthodontist to make braces customized for your teeth. Standard braces are made to fit the average tooth and are predominantly used by orthodontists. Custom braces can be made to match the unique anatomy and shape of your individual teeth. The orthodontist can take an impression or digital scan of your teeth. The lab gets this information and uses it to digitally create brackets to fit your teeth. Then, a robot takes the information and fabricates the appliances. Also, custom archwires can be made that follow the unique shape of your archforms. If desired, the orthodontist can modify the shape of the arches, maybe to broaden them to enhance your smile. Also, the computer setup includes the best place on your tooth to position the bracket. The braces come in special trays that transfer the computer designed bracket placement. The orthodontist adds the adhesive to the brackets and places the tray in your mouth. Once the brackets are glued on your teeth, the trays are removed, and the brackets are on the perfect spot. Using trays to bond brackets to teeth is called indirect bonding. Direct bonding involves the orthodontist individually placing brackets one by one on your teeth.

The benefits of using this technology have been researched. The patients tend to have shorter treatment times and have fewer appointments. The bonding appointment is shorter because of the indirect bonding technique. Custom braces can be made for facial bonding or lingual bonding. Metal and ceramic braces can be made.

Will braces interfere with playing sports?

No. It is recommended, however, that patients protect their smiles by wearing a mouthguard when participating in any sporting activity. Mouthguards are inexpensive, comfortable, and come in a variety of colors and patterns.

Will braces interfere with playing musical instruments?

No. However, there may be an initial period of adjustment. In addition, special covers that fit over the braces can be provided to prevent discomfort to your cheeks and lips.

13

ALTERNATIVES TO BRACES

There are more esthetic options for patients who prefer not to wear braces.

Clear aligners

Some patients want absolutely nothing to show on their teeth at any time, or they don't want the possibility of appliances irritating their cheeks or tongue. Another option for these patients are clear aligners. One example is Invisalign®, but there are other brands that work on the same principle.

Clear aligner treatment uses a series of nearly invisible, removable, and comfortable aligners that no one can tell you're wearing. So, you can smile more during treatment as well as after. Impressions or digital scans are made and sent to the company's lab. The orthodontist prescribes what he wants the aligners to do. The lab sends him a treatment plan that he verifies on the computer. Next, the lab makes the aligners with 3-D computer imaging technology that has been proven effective. You wear each set of aligners for about 2 weeks, removing them only to eat, drink, brush, and floss. As you replace each aligner with the next in the series, your teeth will move —

little by little, week by week — until they have straightened to the final position your orthodontist has prescribed. You must wear these aligners for 22 hours or more each day. It is really important for the patient to be committed and to cooperate with the strict 22 hours rule. Wearing them less or taking breaks can delay treatment or compromise the final result. Sometimes, the orthodontist will bond special engagers to your teeth to facilitate certain tooth movements and hold the aligners better.

Some desired tooth movements are hard to successfully correct with clear aligners. Not everyone is a good candidate for clear aligner treatment. Your orthodontist can tell you if you are a candidate for this mode of treatment.

Why would I want it? Not only are the aligners almost invisible, they are removable, so you can eat and drink what you want while in treatment. Plus, brushing and flossing are no problem. They are also comfortable, with no metal to cause mouth abrasions during treatment. And no metal wires usually means you spend less time in your doctor's office getting adjustments. Figure 13-1 shows a clear aligner both on and off the teeth.

Figure 13-1. Clear aligner, off and on teeth.

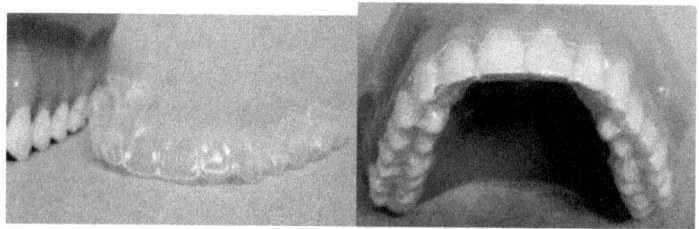

Lingual braces

Another option exists for those patients who don't want

braces to show in their smile, but they may not trust themselves to faithfully wear clear aligners. Braces are placed behind your teeth, on the tongue side, so no one will know that you are wearing braces unless you tell them. With lingual braces you get efficient, effective tooth movement and great esthetics. Almost anyone can wear lingual braces. Lingual braces have been used to treat men and women of any age, but more commonly used with adults. Most people who can be treated with regular braces can be treated with lingual braces, but only your orthodontist can tell you if lingual braces are the right treatment option for you. Some orthodontists chose not to routinely use lingual brackets because the mechanics of treatment are different, and they would prefer to use traditional labial brackets. Figure 13-2 shows lingual braces.

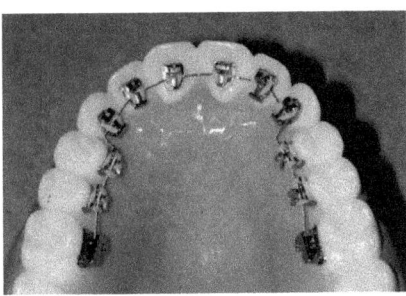

Figure 13-2. Lingual braces.

14

HOW DOES THE ORTHODONTIST PUT BRACES ON MY TEETH?

Braces go on the teeth fairly easily, and bands are just a little more work. There are two methods of bonding brackets, direct bonding and indirect bonding. The key is the orthodontist needs the teeth to be clean, dry, and free from saliva.

Once you are in the chair, the orthodontist or assistant will clean your teeth with a special toothpaste (pumice) similar to what your dentist uses to polish your teeth. The assistant will wash and dry the teeth. Some orthodontists use a retractor, or a tool that holds your lips, cheeks, and tongue away from the teeth. Now that your teeth are clean and dry, a special dental bonding adhesive or cement is used. There may be multiple steps or components to the bonding agent, or he may use a "single-step" adhesive. The orthodontist applies the adhesive to the tooth. Meanwhile an assistant is applying some adhesive to the bracket. The orthodontist will directly place the bracket on the ideal spot on the tooth. Next, the orthodontist will shine an intense blue light on the bracket for a few seconds to cure the adhesive. Now the bracket is bonded to the tooth. The orthodontist will continue the process on the next tooth and directly bond the brackets individually to all the teeth.

Indirect bonding of the teeth is a little different. The orthodontist uses a stone or digital model of your teeth made at the diagnostic records appointment. He places the brackets on the model exactly where he wants them. He will create a transfer tray that holds the brackets in the precise positions and transfers these positions to your mouth. So, on the bonding day for the indirect bonding technique, most of the initial steps are the same. The teeth are cleaned and dried. The orthodontist applies the adhesive to the teeth, and the assistant applies adhesive to the brackets. However, with the indirect method, the transfer tray is placed in your mouth with the brackets in them. The brackets are cured all at once or in big sections. The tray is removed, and the brackets are bonded to the teeth.

Banding teeth is also easy. Each band fits around the tooth, and a snug fit is desired. Separators that were placed about a week ago are removed. There is now a small space around the tooth to allow the thin band to slide around the tooth without hitting the adjacent teeth. The teeth are cleaned. A band is tried on, with the use of a special stick that the patient bites. The biting force helps to push the band around the tooth. Once the desired fit and position of the band is found, the assistant will remove and dry the band. Orthodontic cement will be placed inside the band, and your teeth will be dried. The band with the cement is placed right back around the tooth until the cement is cured. A curing light may not be necessary.

The entire bonding and banding appointments can last from 30 minutes to 90 minutes. This appointment will be on the longer side if top and bottom braces are all put on this day. Since bands have to be fitted, this appointment will be longer if you need bands on your teeth.

Does this hurt? No. The placement of brackets and bands on your teeth does not hurt. You may have to stay open for a while, but that is it. The separators come out with little resistance because there is now a tiny space between the teeth. You will experience some soreness of your teeth a few hours after the braces are bonded and for the next couple of days. The archwires will start to act on the teeth, and the movement process will begin. The soreness will really only be felt when you chew food or squeeze your teeth together. This initial soreness lasts about 2-4 days and will be mild to moderate in intensity. Your lips and cheeks may need one to two weeks to get used to the braces on your teeth.

15

HOW OFTEN DO I HAVE APPOINTMENTS?

Now you have your braces! When do you come back for adjustments?

Orthodontists vary on when you come back for adjustments and how often. Most orthodontists will not ask you to come back for at least 6 weeks after the bonding appointment. Some wait 10 weeks. The first archwires are soft and act over a long time, so you may be able to wait a long time before your first adjustment. You may have to come back sooner for special circumstances. Orthodontists should see you soon if you have a Rapid Maxillary Expander or some other appliances. Some orthodontists would rather change the elastic "O's" or chain over shorter intervals. Some orthodontists may want to just check your hygiene to see how you are cleaning around the braces.

At the next visit, you will most likely have new wires placed and new elastic "O's" tied. On average, you will be asked to come in every 6 weeks for adjustment appointments.

Adjustment appointments usually last 15 to 30 minutes unless extra procedures are indicated. To make updated x-rays, make new appliances, or reposition brackets can add time to your appointment.

Does this hurt? Adjustment appointments themselves
do not hurt. If you get a new archwire or if the
orthodontist adjusts the wire, your teeth may be sore for
2-3 days. Generally, the pain and soreness is mild and
less than right after your braces were put on.

Orthodontic Emergencies

Occasionally, you may have to see the orthodontist for an
"emergency" before your next scheduled visit. With all
the tiny parts that go along with braces, there may be a
time when an archwire is poking you or a bracket is loose.
There are instances when you need to go to the
orthodontist immediately, and other times aren't so
urgent.

True orthodontic emergencies are very rare, but when
they do occur someone at the office should be available
to help you. As a general rule, you should call the office
if you experience severe pain or when you have a painful
appliance problem that you can't take care of yourself.
You might be surprised to learn that you may be able to
temporarily solve many problems yourself until you
schedule an appointment with the office. Allowing your
appliance to remain damaged for an extended period of
time may result in disruptions in your treatment plan.

Loose Wire: Using tweezers, try to put your wire back
into place. If doing this and using wax doesn't help, as a
last resort use a small fingernail clipper which has been
cleaned with alcohol to clip the wire behind the last tooth
to which it is securely fastened. If your discomfort
continues, place wax on it.

Lost separator: Call the office. You may or may not have
to go back to the office for a new separator to be placed.
If one falls out and you don't call, it may be more difficult

to find the best fitting band for that tooth.

Loose bracket or band: If your bracket or band is still attached to the wire, you should leave it in place and put wax on it. If the bracket comes out entirely, wrap the bracket with a tissue. Call the office to schedule a visit, and bring the bracket with you.

Loose bonded retainer: If your appliance is poking you, place wax on the offending part of your appliance. Call the office to schedule a visit.

Loose removable retainer: If it needs to be adjusted or tightened, call the office to schedule an appointment. Try to wear it in the meantime, unless it absolutely cannot stay in place.

Headgear does not fit: Sometimes headgear discomfort is caused by not wearing the headgear as instructed by your orthodontist. Please refer to the instructions provided by your orthodontist. If the facebow is bent, please call the office for assistance. Surprisingly, the headgear may hurt less as it's worn more, so be sure you're getting in the prescribed hours.

General soreness: When you get your braces on, you may feel general soreness in your mouth, and teeth may be tender to biting pressures for three to five days. Placing Orabase on the affected area may help; this can be found in most pharmacies. If the tenderness is severe, take acetaminophen or any non-aspirin pain relievers that you normally would take for headache or similar pain. Check with your orthodontist for instructions for dose and frequency of the medication. Take only as prescribed by your orthodontist. The lips, cheeks, and tongue may also become irritated for one to two weeks as they toughen and become accustomed to the surface of the braces. You can put wax on the braces to lessen this discomfort.

<u>Loose spring (bite corrector)</u>: Call the office for advice. If any parts come completely off the braces, hold on to them and bring them with you to the office when you return.

<u>Loose elastic "O" or chain</u>: Call the office to determine what the next step is. Sometimes you can wait until your next scheduled visit.

<u>Wire poking or sticking</u>: Call the office to talk you through the next step. Small wires can be shifted away from the poking side. Grab the wire with tweezers and pull the wire to slide it away from the long, irritated side. If teeth have moved or spaces closed since your last visit, the wire may have become longer since your last visit, and you will probably have to go to the office for the wire to be clipped.

16

WHY DO I HAVE TO WEAR RUBBER BANDS?

The job of the braces and the archwires is to get the teeth straight and aligned. Orthodontists have another tool to help the teeth fit together better and close spaces between teeth. Rubber bands, or elastics, help the teeth to come together and improve your smile. There are many different ways they can be hooked up to your braces. Your orthodontist will determine the correct configuration to wear in order to move the teeth efficiently.

Smaller overjets (Class II) can be corrected with rubber bands. These elastics will pull the lower incisors forward to meet the upper incisors. Small underbite tendencies (Class III) can be treated with elastics that pull the upper incisors forward. Open bites can be treated with elastics that pull the upper and lower teeth together. Some posterior crossbites can also be corrected with elastics. Pictures of some elastics being worn can be found in Chapter 19.

Elastics must be worn nearly 24 hours per day to be effective and move the teeth. The only times you may not have to wear them is during eating and brushing. If you don't wear them as instructed by your orthodontist, your smile will not be as beautiful as it can be, and your time in treatment will be longer that it has to be. Also, your orthodontist may decide to use some device, like a spring, that attaches to your braces and that you cannot remove.

Does this hurt? Rubber bands can make your teeth sore. This lasts about 2-3 days after starting to wear them, and it is mild to moderate in intensity. The soreness is similar to changing an archwire or doing an archwire adjustment. The key is to continue to wear them without taking breaks. Each time you take an elastic vacation and re-start, the soreness comes back. Wearing the elastics continuously without breaks eliminates the soreness, except the initial 2 days after first getting them.

17

DO I STILL HAVE TO SEE MY REGULAR DENTIST WHILE I HAVE MY BRACES?

Yes, Yes, and Yes. You need to see your regular dentist while you have braces for cleanings and checkups. In fact, some patients will be advised to see their dentist more often than usual, maybe every 3 or 4 months instead of twice a year.

Braces and archwires act like food traps. They are obstacles to keeping your teeth clean and spotless. With a little extra care and time, nearly all patients can keep their teeth clean. A few patients will have some plaque build up. Seeing your dentist and hygienist ensures that the plaque not stay on the teeth for too long and not start any decay around the brackets.

Dentists also have tools that the orthodontist doesn't have to look for cavities between the teeth. It is essential to keep your regular dentist visits to catch any cavities early as they develop.

Adult patients with previous periodontal disease should see their regular dentist or periodontist every 3 or 4 months while they have braces. The dentist or periodontist will measure and assess how the health of the gums and bone that supports the teeth progresses during treatment.

18

WHAT ARE PHASE I AND PHASE II TREATMENTS?

Phase I or Early Treatment

Phase I, or early interceptive treatment, is limited orthodontic treatment (i.e. expander, partial braces, headgear, functional appliances) started before all of the permanent teeth have erupted. Such treatment can occur between the ages of six and ten. Extraction of baby teeth can be recommended to make room for erupting permanent teeth. Space maintainers can be used to prevent space loss and extra crowding when baby teeth are lost too early. Early treatment is sometimes recommended to make more space for developing teeth, correction of crossbites, overbites, underbites, or harmful oral habits. The majority of children do not need Phase I treatment. Early treatment is indicated in severe cases that need intervention immediately to prevent impaction of teeth and eruption problems, to improve severe bite problems, and to initiate jaw growth modification in patients with jaw growth discrepancies.

The timing of early treatment is important as the orthodontist utilizes certain growth spurts to modify growth and the eruption of teeth; waiting until teenage years would lose this important window of time. Goals of early treatment are limited to correcting the major problems. The final result is not a perfect occlusion; changes in growth and eruption of remaining teeth affect the outcome. It usually lasts 12 to 18 months. Early treatment does not eliminate the need for orthodontic treatment later. In fact, most children who require early treatment will also need comprehensive treatment as a teen. Early treatment reduces the severity of the orthodontic problem that otherwise would not be able to be predictably corrected in one phase later on. Early treatment may be started for less severe problems when there is teasing at school and psychosocial concerns.

Posterior crossbites can be corrected with expanders that fit on the top teeth. Rapid Maxillary Expanders (RME) can be banded to molars and have a special key that fits into the screw (Figure 18-1). A parent or older sibling actually turns the screw to activate the expansion. This can be either fast (rapid) or slow expansion. RME's are also known as RPE's (Rapid Palatal Expanders) and can actually widen the entire maxillary bone structure. Another appliance for upper arch expansion is a W-arch (similar to a quad helix) that can be banded to molars (Figure 18-2). There is no screw or key to turn. These are typically gentler and act over a longer periods of time. Arms can extend forward and help move front teeth.

Does this hurt? You can expect your teeth to be sore for about a day after the first few turns of the RPE screw. The soreness is mild. After that, there is a pressure that is felt for a few minutes after turning the screw. Getting used to eating and talking with the appliance is fairly quick, and most kids function normally after 3-5 days. With the W-arch, the child's teeth may feel sore after initial placement and later activations for a couple of days. Again, the soreness is mild. It takes about 3-5 days for the kids to get used to eating and talking with it.

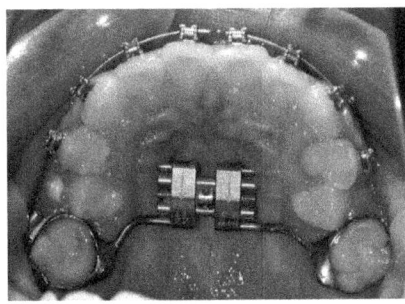

Figure18-1. Rapid Maxillary Expander on top teeth with bands on the molars. Metal braces are bonded to the other teeth.

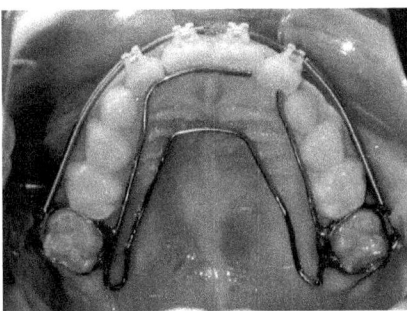

Figure 18-2. W-arch used to expand the maxillary arch, banded to molars. An anterior arm helps to move front teeth. Clear braces are bonded to the front teeth.

Growth modification can be started to help guide the growth of the jaws in kids with skeletal overbites or underbites. There are many appliances that are designed for this kind of treatment, and they fall into two categories: removable functional appliances and fixed functional appliances. Removable appliances allow the patient to take them out of their mouths to eat and brush. Fixed appliances are cemented into place, and only the orthodontist can remove it.

Large overjets and overbites are associated with Class II bites where the lower jaw is too small. A removable appliance such as an Activator (Figure 18-3) or Twin Block treats this malocclusion. An acrylic appliance is made to have the patient bite down and hold his lower jaw forward. It attaches to the teeth with tiny metal clasps. Sometimes, a metal wire is used on the front teeth for stability. The appliance is designed to guide the growth of the lower jaw forward. Also, the upper incisors lean back, and the lower incisors lean forward.

Another famous removable appliance is the headgear. Headgears come in three varieties: two treat Class II patients and one is for Class III patients (Figure 18-4). Headgears work on modifying the growth of the maxilla. Cervical pull (neck strap) headgear uses bands on the maxillary molars, and the bands have a special tube that fits the inner bow of the facebow (Figure 18-5). The outer bow of the facebow attaches to a strap that fits around the back of the neck below the ears. This slows the growth of the upper jaw and pushes the upper teeth straight back. The high-pull (head cap) headgear has a strap that fits around the top of your head, above your ears. The facebow and molar band tubes are the same as the cervical pull headgear. This also slows the growth of the upper jaw and moves the upper jaw and teeth back and up. Class III, underbite malocclusions are treated with a reverse-pull headgear. The reverse-pull headgear uses a special "mask" or bar that fits against the front of your face, usually resting against the forehead and chin. Bands are fitted around molars and are usually attached to a special appliance like an expander. Elastic rubber bands are attached to the top teeth and connect to the facemask. This pulls the top teeth and top jaw forward (Figure 18-6).

For removable appliance therapy to be successful, they should be worn as much as possible. Also, consistent wear is needed, and weeklong breaks should be avoided. These must be worn to work. More than 12 hours per day is desirable. All day would be great! However orthodontists know that they are difficult to wear to school and while playing with friends. It is recommended that they not be worn while playing sports or during any kind of horseplay with friends.

Does this hurt? No. Children get used to these appliances fairly quickly and complain very little of pain. There is some adjustment to having the bulky appliances in their mouths, especially during sleep. Most kids feel like it is normal after about 2 weeks. Soreness from the rubber bands on the reverse-pull headgear may last 3-5 days after starting the appliance, but is generally mild.

Figure 18-3. An Activator for growth modification.

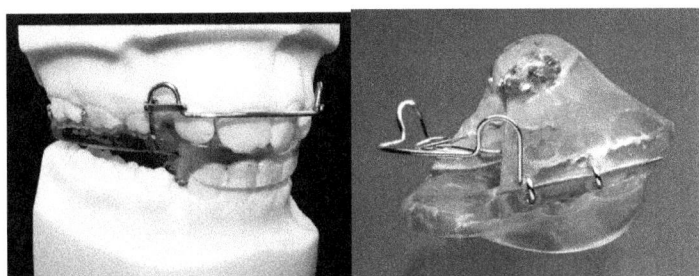

Figure 18-4. The different kinds of headgear used for growth modification.

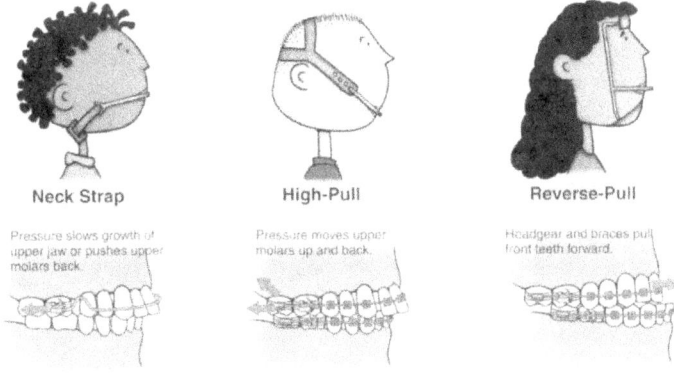

Neck Strap

Pressure slows growth of upper jaw or pushes upper molars back.

High-Pull

Pressure moves upper molars up and back.

Reverse-Pull

Headgear and braces pull front teeth forward.

Figure 18-5. A facebow used with cervical pull and high-pull headgear.

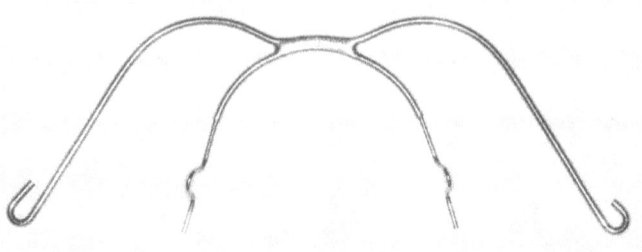

Figure 18-6. Reverse pull headgear

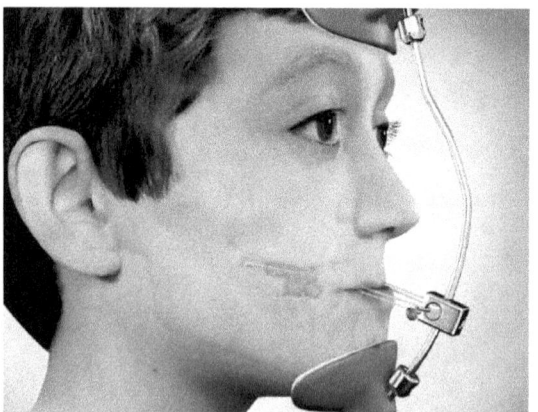

A Herbst appliance is an example of a fixed functional appliance used for Class II growth modification (Figure 18-7). There are many designs and variations of a Herbst, but essentially there are crowns or bands that fit around upper and lower molars. Rigid arms connect the upper and lower crowns and force the patient to bite with the lower jaw going forward. The orthodontist activates the appliances to move the lower jaw forward in increments. Don't be alarmed if the child looks like he has an underbite. The orthodontist usually prefers to "over-correct" the bite, as some relapse will occur once the appliance is removed. Braces on the front teeth may or may not be used. The appliance moves the upper incisors back and the lower incisors forward. There is a skeletal benefit also, as the lower jaw is guided forward. The advantage of this appliance is that it is worn 24 hours a day, and you don't have to rely on the child to follow instructions for wearing. However, there may be extra appointments, as there tends to be some breakage of the parts. These stay cemented in the child's mouth for 9-14 months.

Does this hurt? As scary as it looks, this doesn't cause much pain. It feels awkward when the child eats and talks because it takes time to get used to the forward position of the lower jaw. It takes about 5-7 days to function like normal. Teeth don't really get sore, unless braces are used on the front teeth. That soreness lasts 2-3 days after initial placement and subsequent activations. Rarely, the arms cause irritation to the inside of the child's cheeks.

Figure 18-7. Herbst appliance for growth modification.

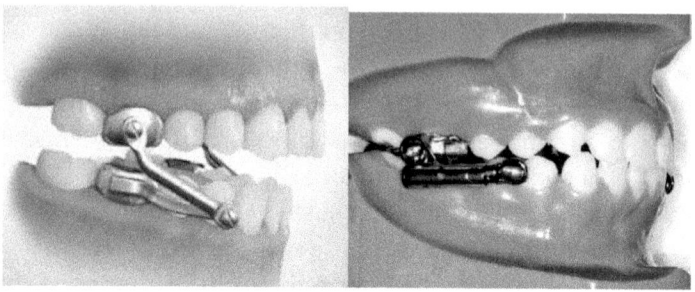

If no early treatment with orthodontic appliances is necessary, your orthodontist may recommend extractions of baby teeth to make room for erupting permanent teeth. This can help guide the permanent teeth to the correct positions. **Serial extraction** treatment or **guidance of eruption** is treatment used when there is moderate to severe crowding. Baby teeth are removed at certain times and sequences to guide the permanent teeth into the arch. If there is too much crowding, then permanent teeth may have to be removed to make room for the remaining teeth. Figure 18-8A shows a patient with crowding in both arches and anterior crossbites. The only treatment performed was extraction of four baby teeth. Spontaneous alignment of the remaining teeth and correction of the crossbite were completed (Figure 18-8B).

Does this hurt? Baby teeth extractions are generally quick and easy procedures with little pain afterwards. Children can usually return to school the same day as the procedure. Your general dentist most often does the extractions and will make sure the child is numb and comfortable. Parents are surprised to see how long the roots of some of these baby teeth can be!

Figure 18-8A

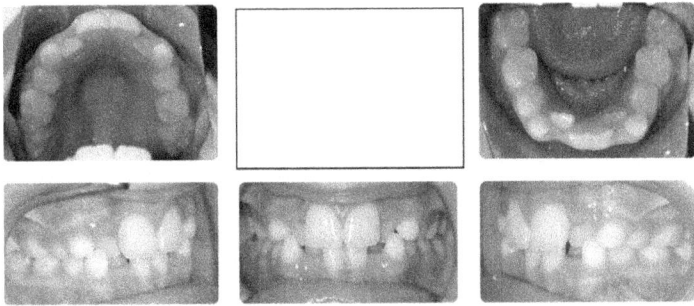

Figure 18-8B

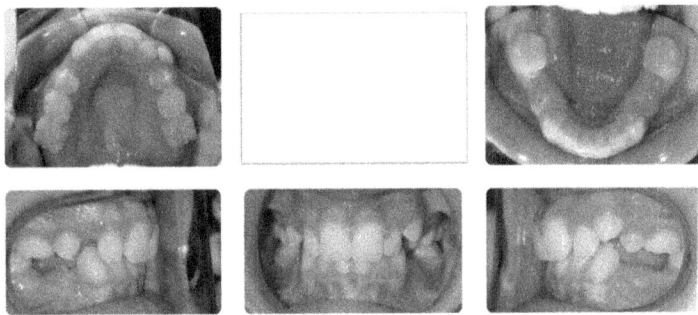

Sometimes a **space maintainer** will be required to prevent the other teeth from moving into the space needed for erupting teeth when crowding is present (Figure 18-9). Space maintainers are taken out just as the desired teeth begin to erupt.

Does this hurt? No, space maintainers do not hurt and generally do not get in the way of eating or talking.

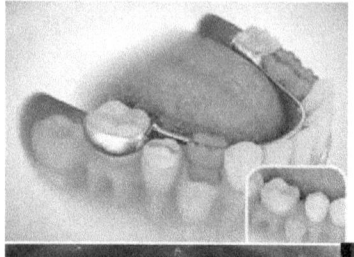

Figure 18-9. Space maintainers on the lower teeth and upper teeth.

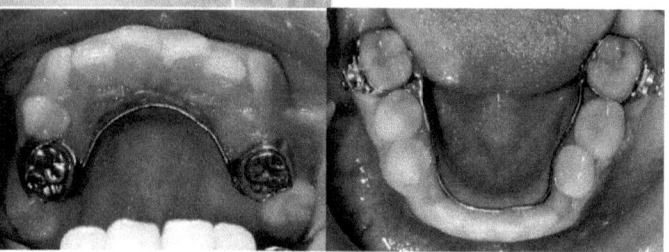

Before bands, crowns, Herbst appliances, or space maintainers are delivered, a tiny space needs to be opened between the teeth where bands will be cemented. Separators (Figure 18-10) are placed between these teeth to open the contact and allow the thin metal of the band to slide between those teeth. Separators are inserted and stay in place for about a week before the band fitting appointment. Separators are tiny elastic "O" rings that actually move the teeth a tiny bit. For tighter contacts, metal separators with a different shape can be used.

Figure 18-10. Separators inserted between teeth before banding.

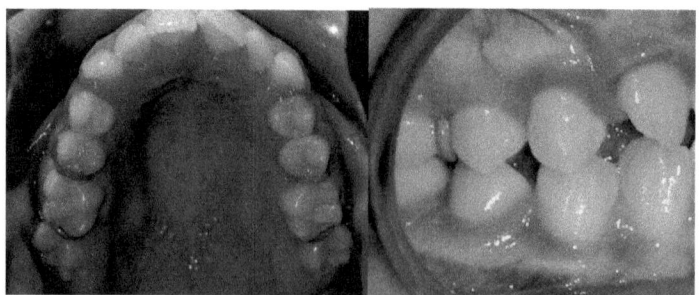

Does this hurt? Ok, let's be honest. Separators do make most people sore for a couple of days. Younger kids complain less, and older kids complain more. Adults are mixed. You can feel these when you bite; it feels like you have a piece of meat or some food stuck between your teeth when you chew. Separators are considered the most "painful" part of braces. The good news is that it doesn't last a long time, and it gets easier from here.

Finger sucking habits that persist past age six should be stopped as soon as they are discovered. Prolonged sucking of the thumb or fingers can lead to protrusion of the upper incisors, a narrow upper arch, posterior crossbite, and anterior open bite. These habits can be hard to break for some kids. Many want to stop, but they just can't do it. To make matters worse, some children suck their fingers in their sleep and have no control over this subconscious habit. An appliance designed to help break the persistent habit can be made to fit on the upper arch. These should not be removable. An example of a finger habit appliance is in Figure 18-11.

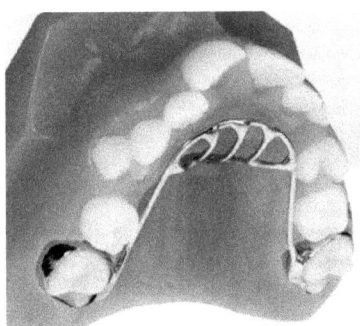

Figure 18-11. An appliance used to stop persistent finger or thumb sucking.

Does this hurt? No, finger habit appliances do not hurt and are well tolerated by kids. It takes only a couple of days to get used to eating and talking with it.

Samples of early treatments are highlighted below.

Figures 18-12A and 18-12B are the before and after treatment photos of a patient with a severe anterior open bite. A small midline diastema was present. Upper and lower braces were bonded to the incisors. Vertical elastics were worn from the top incisors to the bottom incisors to close the open bite. Also, tongue trainers were bonded to the upper incisors on the lingual side (Figure18-12A) to control a tongue thrust habit. Also, notice the ankylosed, submerged lower primary first molars; these are the fourth teeth from the middle.

Figure 18-12A

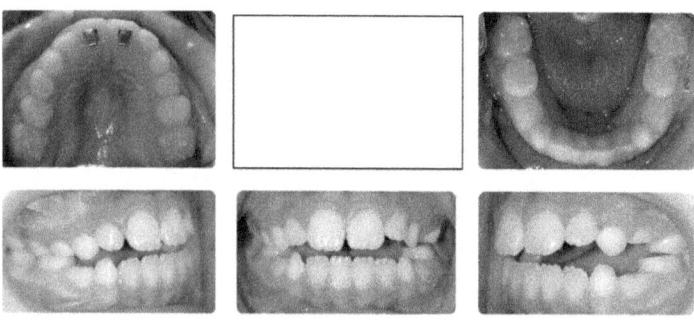

Figure 18-12B

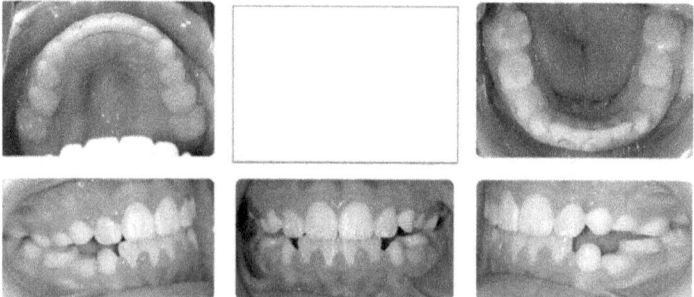

Figures 18-13A and 18-13B are the before and after photos of a patient with an anterior crossbite, deep bite, crowding, and blocked out maxillary lateral incisors. Braces on the top teeth only were used with coil springs on the archwire to correct the crossbite and make room for the blocked out teeth.

Figure 18-13A

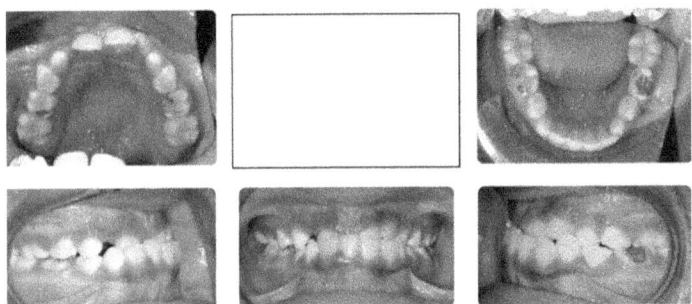

Figure 18-13B

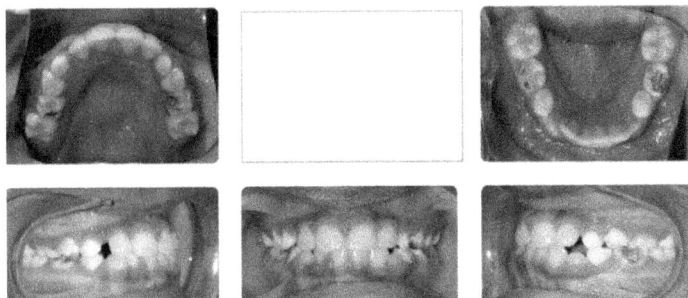

Figures 18-14A and 18-14B are the before and after photos of a patient with crowding, anterior crossbite, and recession. Metal braces were bonded in the upper and lower arches.

Figure 18-14A

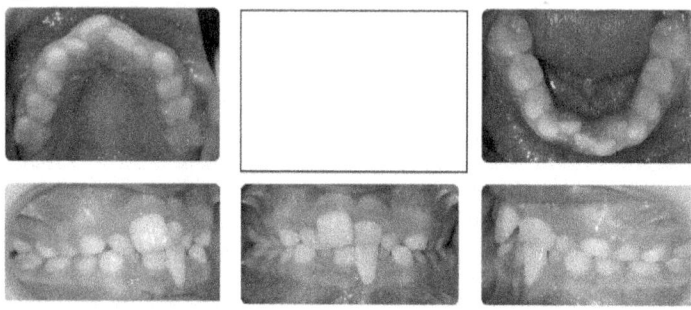

Figure 18-14B

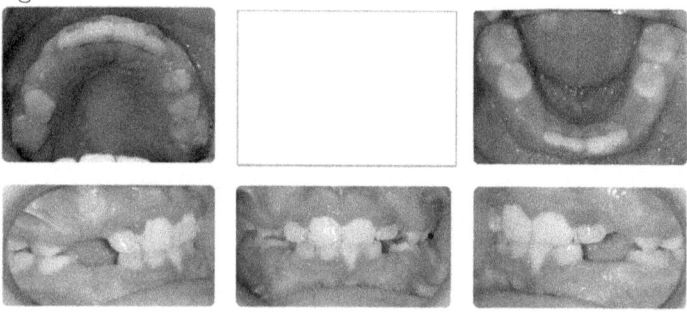

Figures 18-15A and 18-15B are the before and after photos of a patient with an anterior open bite, protrusive upper incisors (Class II), and maxillary spacing. Braces were bonded to the upper and lower teeth. Elastic chain was used to close the upper spaces. A high-pull headgear was introduced midway through the treatment and continued after the front braces were removed.

Figure 18-15A

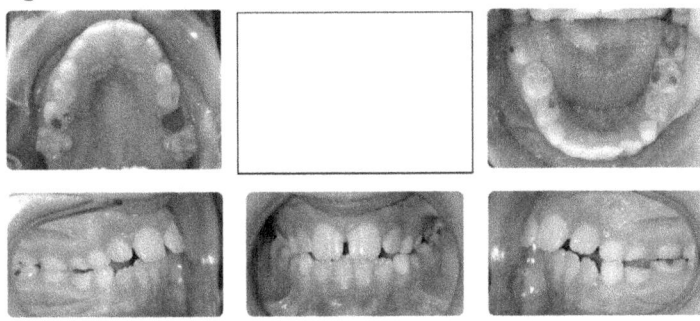

Figure 18-15B

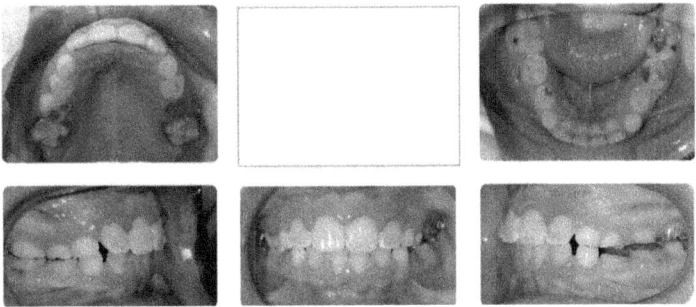

Figures 18-16A and 18-16B are before and after photos of a patient with crowding, midline diastema, and blocked out maxillary lateral incisors. Upper and lower braces were bonded and coil springs were used to open space for the blocked out teeth and push the upper front teeth together.

Figure 18-16A

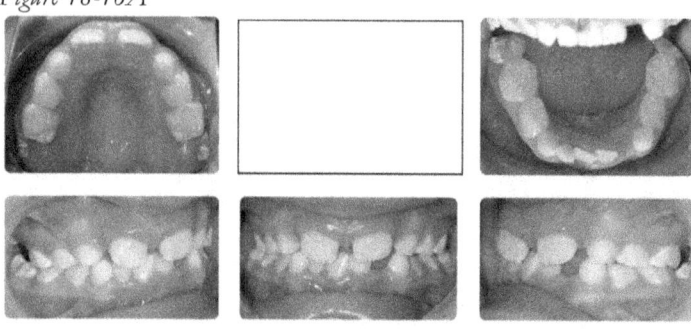

Figure 18-16B

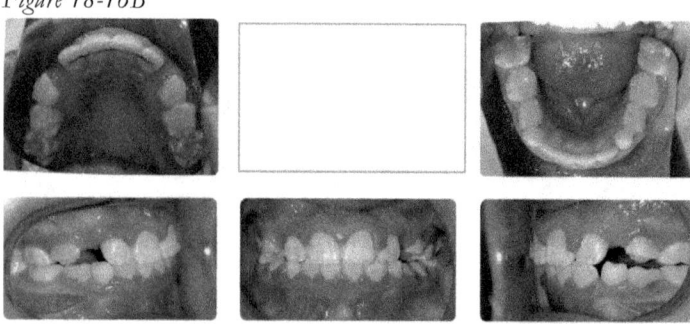

Figures 18-17A, 18-17B and 18-17C are before, during, and after photos of a patient with upper and lower crowding, deep bite, midline discrepancy (lower off to the patient's right), and blocked out teeth on the patient's lower right. Braces were bonded to upper and lower teeth. Coil spring was used to open the space on the lower right to allow the permanent teeth to erupt. The midline was corrected, and the deep bite improved.

Figure 18-17A

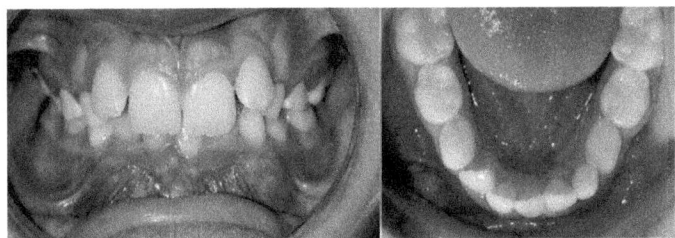

Figure 18-17B

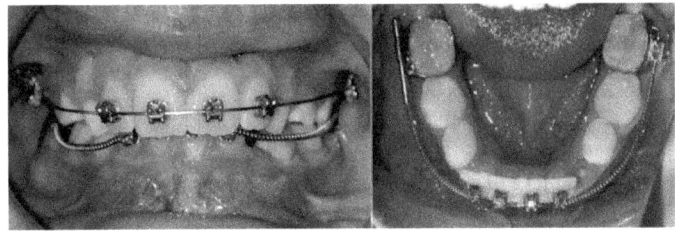

Figure 18-17C

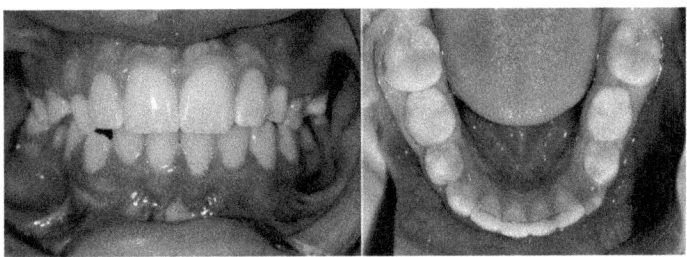

Phase II Treatment or Second Phase Treatment

Phase II treatment is also called comprehensive treatment because it involves full braces when all of the permanent teeth have erupted, usually between the ages of eleven and thirteen. This follows Phase I treatment and allows for full correction of all the permanent teeth. A second phase of treatment is usually needed after an early phase, as problems that exist at an early age tend to manifest as the other permanent teeth erupt. Phase II treatment usually last 12-18 months.

The following are examples of patients who had Phase I and Phase II treatment, also called multiphase treatment.

Figures 18-18A and 18-18B are photos of a patient who had protrusive incisors, slightly protrusive lips, a Class II bite, and maxillary spacing. Early treatment used top and bottom braces to align the teeth, decrease the protrusiveness of the upper incisors, and close the midline diastema. Phase II started and all the teeth were bonded with brackets. Class II correcting springs and elastics were used to correct the bite.

Figure 18-18A

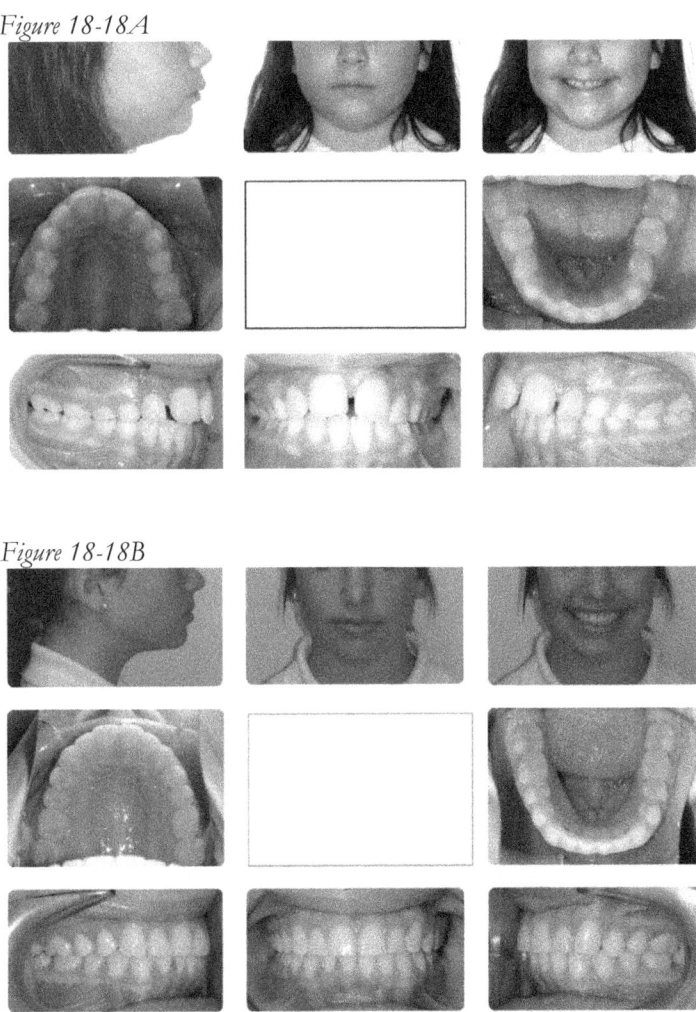

Figure 18-18B

Figures 18-19A and 18-19B are photos of a patient who had a Class II bite, maxillary spacing, small lower jaw, and deep bite. Early treatment used top and bottom braces to close the spaces and improve the deep bite. A cervical pull headgear was used for growth modification and Class II correction. Phase II started when all the permanent teeth were erupted. All teeth were bonded with brackets and elastics were used to improve the bite.

Figure 18-19A

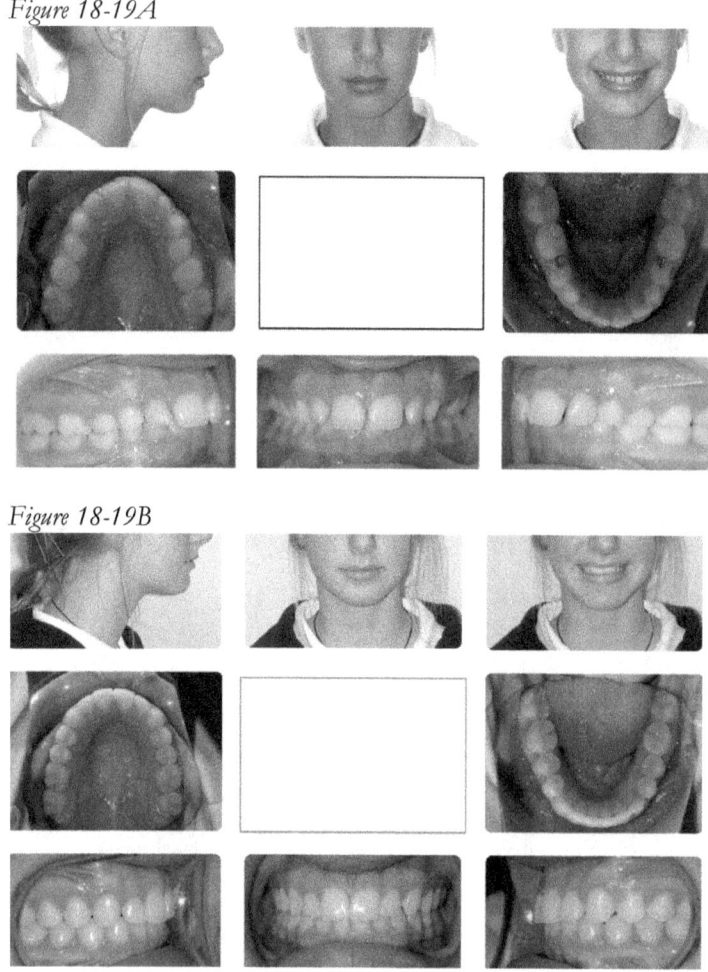

Figure 18-19B

Figure 18-20 shows a deep bite with wear on the lower incisors. Phase I and Phase II treatment were completed to correct the deep bite.

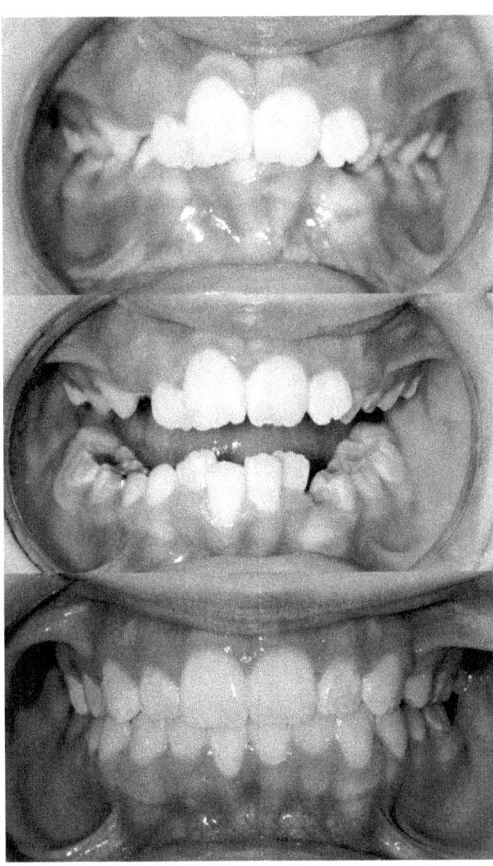

Figure 18-20. Deep bite with wear on the lower incisors. The deep bite was corrected after Phase I and Phase II treatment.

19

WHAT IS COMPREHENSIVE TREATMENT, OR SINGLE PHASE TREATMENT?

Most children will not need to start early phase treatment and will benefit from starting treatment when all of the permanent teeth are erupted. Single phase, comprehensive treatment is orthodontic therapy that aims to achieve all or most of the possible goals of orthodontics described previously in this book. So, most teenagers and adults fall into this category. All malocclusions are addressed, and all or most teeth will have brackets on them. The appendix at the end of this book shows before and after photos of a few examples of common cases treated with different single phase treatment plans.

Some of the appliances used in early treatment can be used in the single phase treatment. Rapid Maxillary Expanders (RME's) (Figure 19-1) and Herbst appliances (Figure 19-2) can be used at the same time as the braces.

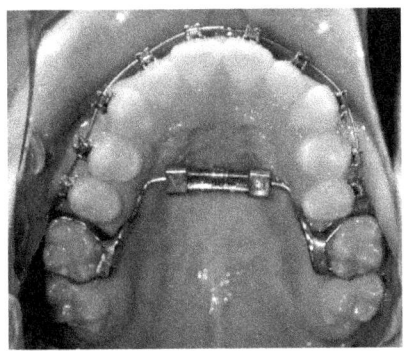

Figure 19-1. Rapid Maxillary Expander used in single phase treatment along with braces.

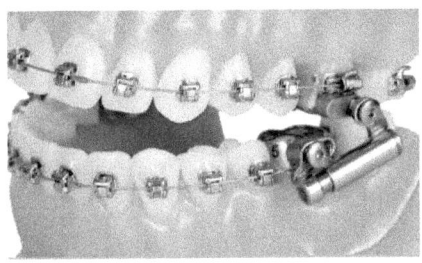

Figure 19-2. Herbst type appliance used with braces in single phase treatment.

Does this hurt? The expanders don't cause much discomfort, even though they sound like they would. Some pressure is felt for a few minutes after the key is turned, but the pressure goes away pretty quickly. A few days are needed to get used to eating and talking with the appliance. Herbst appliances will cause some mild discomfort for 2-3 days after you get it. It will take 5-7 days to get used to talking and eating with a Herbst appliance. Rarely, cheek irritation can happen until the cheeks get used to having the appliance there.

The Herbst is used to correct overjet and Class II problems. Other appliances used to fix big overjets include some kind of spring that connects to the braces and pushes the lower teeth forward. These springs and the Herbst appliances have the benefit of staying in the mouth 24 hours per day, and they don't require the patient's cooperation with wearing them as asked. Figure 19-3 shows an example of a Class II corrector spring.

Does this hurt? These springs can cause some mild to moderate soreness of your teeth for 2-4 days after placement. It causes just a little more soreness than regular archwire adjustments. Some irritation of the cheeks can occur for a few days until the cheeks get used to having the appliance there.

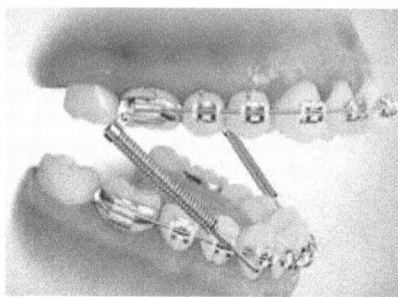

Figure 19-3. An example of a Class II correcting spring.

Elastics, or rubber bands, are also used in comprehensive therapy to correct different types of bite problems. There are many different ways to hook these to your braces, and the orthodontist can modify the exact configuration. Elastics can be placed and removed by the patient. Again, if the patient does not cooperate with wearing the elastics, the desired results won't happen. The orthodontist may decide to use a Herbst or a spring corrector when he sees the patient not wearing the elastics as advised. Typically, rubber bands must be worn 24 hours per day, except when eating or brushing. Patients should definitely wear them at night. Your orthodontist may modify the time that you wear them depending on your bite. Class II elastics (Figure 19-4) are worn to fix big overjets. Class III elastics (Figure 19-5) are worn to correct underbite problems and pull the upper teeth forward. Vertical elastics (Figure 19-6) are worn to fix open bites. Cross-bite elastics (Figure 19-7) help to correct cross-bites. Special "hooks" on brackets or posts on archwires that look like antennae are used to secure elastics. Elastics also help to correct midline discrepancies and close spaces between teeth.

Does this hurt? Rubber bands can make your teeth sore. This lasts about 2-3 days after starting to wear them, and it is mild to moderate in intensity. The soreness is similar to changing an archwire or doing an archwire adjustment. The key is to continue to wear them without taking breaks. Each time you take an elastic vacation and re-start, the soreness comes back. Wearing the elastics continuously without breaks eliminates the soreness, except the initial 2 days after first getting them.

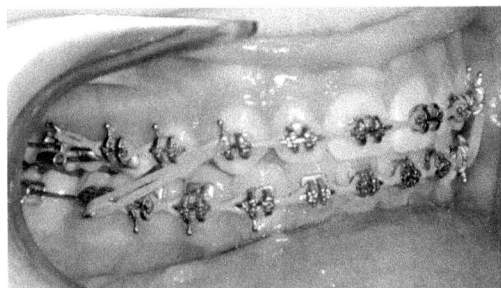

Figure 19-4. Class II elastics pull the lower incisors forward.

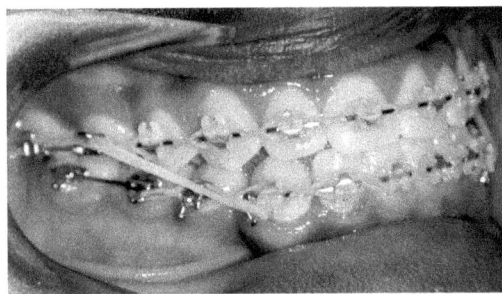

Figure 19-5. Class III elastics pull the upper incisors forward.

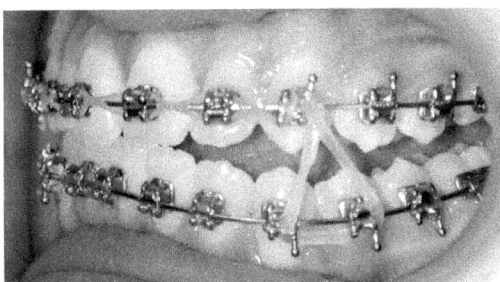

Figure 19-6. Vertical elastics close open bites.

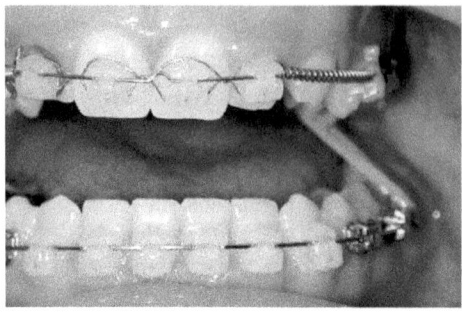

Figure 19-7. Cross-elastics from the lingual of the upper molar to the buccal of the lower molar.

Extractions

Most of the time, the orthodontist puts the braces on, and the teeth will align. However, in some cases, there is just too much crowding to properly align all the teeth present. It is as if the teeth are too big for the jaws. Alignment of severe crowding can lead to teeth that protrude, gingival recession problems, teeth that don't fit as well as they could, and smiles that look too "toothy." One way to make space to accommodate the teeth in a healthy and attractive way is to extract some teeth. Your orthodontist will send you to your dentist to have the teeth removed at the right time. Orthodontic treatment with extractions can lead to more upright incisors and more stable results in some cases.

Usually, in cases with severe crowing and good bites, four permanent teeth are extracted. These four teeth are towards the back of the mouth and are called premolars or bicuspids. The teeth will be aligned, and the remaining extraction space will be closed with the braces. There won't be any gaps left when the braces are removed.

There are also other teeth that can be removed depending on the specific malocclusion. For moderate crowding in the lower arch with a good bite, one lower incisor can be removed. This is more common in adults. For cases with symmetry issues or midlines that don't match, one or three teeth can be extracted. Also, the four teeth extracted don't have to be the exact corresponding teeth in each quadrant. For big overjets (Class II) or protrusive upper incisors, extraction of two upper premolars may be indicated to upright the upper incisors and bring them back to meet the lower incisors. For mild underbites (Class III), extraction of two lower premolars may be indicated to pull the lower incisors behind the upper incisors. In cases where there doesn't look like there is any crowding, four teeth may be extracted if the incisors look too protrusive and the patient has to "strain" his lips around his teeth to make his lips touch.

There are many different extraction patterns, and the orthodontist will base his decision on your specific malocclusion, using the information he gathered at the diagnostic records appointment.

Most patients do not require extractions for their orthodontic treatment.

Does this hurt? Especially in children, extraction of permanent teeth doesn't cause a lot of pain. Most kids don't even report soreness the next day. The dentist usually takes out these teeth fairly easily and quickly. The orthodontic treatment then progresses and feels like treatment in non-extraction cases.

Interproximal Reduction (IPR)

Sometimes there is a lot of crowding, but the orthodontist prefers not to extract teeth. To prevent the teeth becoming protrusive and leaning too far forward, the orthodontist may decide to make some space in a different manner.

Interproximal reduction (IPR) is a way to create some space. The desired teeth are made more slender by reshaping the contacts between some teeth. This could be done with an abrasive disc or a special strip of floss that acts like sandpaper. Usually, only a fraction of a millimeter of enamel is removed from each side of the tooth. Removing this small amount of enamel does not expose the sensitive part of the teeth (dentin) and is painless. The tiny spaces are made then later closed.

Other indications for IPR (also known as ARS or "stripping") include midline adjustments. The orthodontist measures the widths of the teeth before treatment. There is a special formula or ratio of the sizes of the teeth in each arch when compared with each other in an occlusion that fits well. If the upper teeth are too big then there will be too much overjet when the teeth are straight. If the lower teeth are too wide then the lower incisors may not fit behind the upper teeth properly or lead to spacing between the upper incisors. If it is determined that the sizes of the lower teeth are too large relative to the upper teeth, then the orthodontist can slenderize the lower teeth to make them more narrow, fit properly behind the upper incisors, and prevent spaces between the upper incisors.

Does this hurt? No. Slenderizing the teeth is quick and painless. The teeth may feel cold while the orthodontist uses the disc or drill. Your gum tissue may feel like it is temporarily pinched while the orthodontist reshapes the teeth close to the gumline. The teeth shouldn't be sensitive as only a small amount of enamel is being removed.

Impacted Teeth

Impacted teeth are teeth that cannot erupt into the mouth because something is preventing them from doing so. There may not be enough room for the tooth to get to its correct position. The tooth may be growing at a wrong angle or in the wrong direction (ectopic eruption). A baby tooth may be over-retained and deflecting the path of eruption. The gum tissue may be too fibrous and tough to allow the tooth to break through the tissue.

Impacted teeth (Figures 19-8 and 19-9) can be brought into their correct position in the mouth with orthodontic treatment. Another procedure done by an oral surgeon or periodontist may be needed additionally. Usually the braces are started to align the teeth. Space is made to accommodate the impacted tooth. Then, the oral surgeon or periodontist does a little surgery to expose the impacted tooth. Sometimes the exposure and gum tissue removal is enough to allow the tooth to erupt on its own. The orthodontist may prefer to bond a special bracket and chain to the impacted tooth. The orthodontist will attach an elastic or spring to the chain to guide it to its correct position.

Less severe impactions may not require a visit to the oral surgeon. If the impacted tooth isn't far from the arch and if only gum tissue is impeding the eruption, then the orthodontist may use a laser to remove the tissue. This can be done without a shot, just topical anesthetic gel. The procedure only takes a couple of minutes. Enough tissue is removed to bond an attachment or bracket (Figure 19-10).

While we are discussing impacted teeth, let's mention wisdom teeth. Wisdom teeth are also referred to as third molars. They are the teeth that develop behind twelve-year-molars. Most often, there isn't enough room for them to erupt, and they are usually impacted. The dentist or orthodontist will see them on an x-ray, and he may recommend extracting them. Wisdom teeth left impacted or partially erupted can cause some problems, which can be avoided with extractions. They can impinge the roots of the twelve-year-molars, causing damage to those teeth. Very commonly periodontal problems can begin around the twelve-year-molars, causing pain, inflammation, and swelling around these teeth. If the wisdom teeth do partially erupt, it is very difficult to properly clean them because they are so hard to reach. If not cleaned properly, they will decay or harbor more plaque that causes inflammation.

Figure 19-8. Ectopically erupting and impacted maxillary canines. The baby canines were extracted. The permanent canines were exposed and a gold chain was bonded. The chain was attached with elastic thread and brought into the arch.

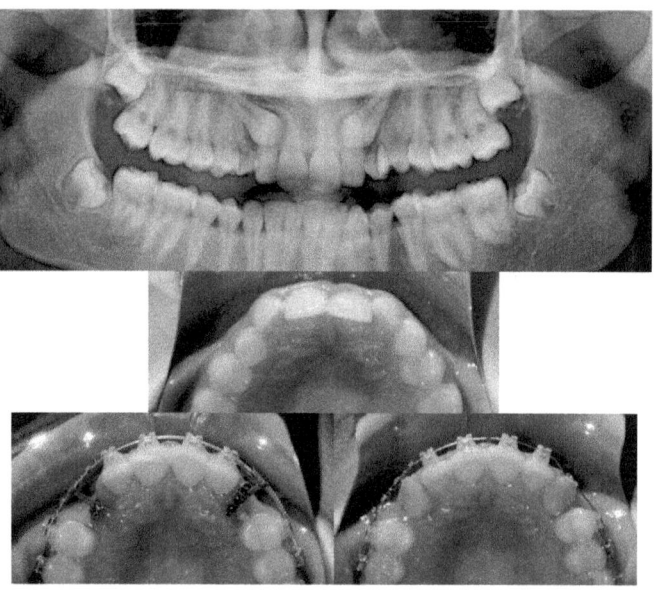

Figure 19-9. Impacted lower second and third molars. The second molar was uprighted and incorporated into the arch.

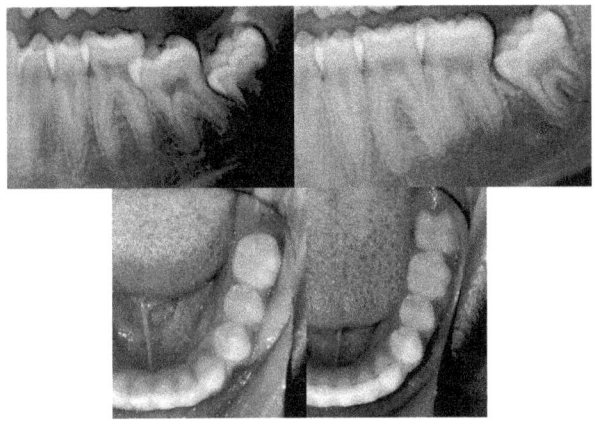

Figure 19-10. Impacted maxillary canine. The soft tissue was removed with a laser. A bracket was bonded and the canine brought to the correct position.

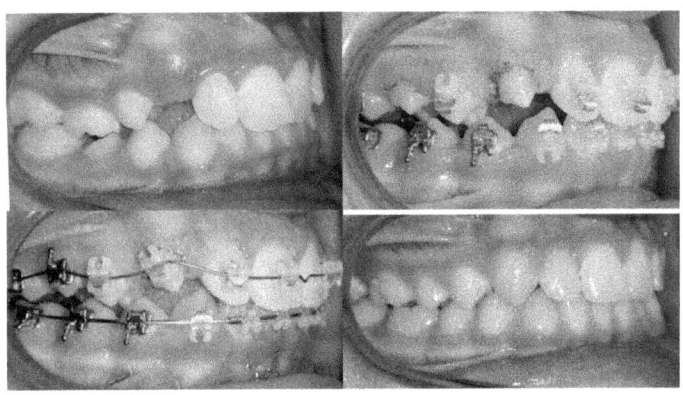

Does this hurt? The exposure procedure may leave the patient with a little discomfort, but it is usually gone by the next day. The adjustments done by the orthodontist will introduce a little soreness and pressure to the impacted tooth that goes away after 1-2 days. During the orthodontic visit, there may be some tenderness in the gums as the elastic is tightened, due to the gum tissue's healing around the chain and being pulled.

Ectopic Eruption

Ectopic eruption can happen when the tooth's movement follows a path uncharacteristic to that specific tooth. Treatment is usually aimed at getting the tooth back on track. Baby or permanent teeth can be extracted. Early treatment with braces or a removable appliance can correct the path of the tooth's eruption.

Does this hurt? This feels like any other orthodontic treatment. If it goes untreated, the ectopic tooth can cause damage to the adjacent teeth, which usually is painless.

Transposed Teeth

Each tooth in your mouth has a specific place it's supposed to occupy. Transposed teeth are teeth that swap places. If a canine is in front of an incisor, there is a transposition.

Transpositions can be fixed by moving the teeth to the correct positions (Figure 19-11). Sometimes moving the teeth can compromise the health of the bone and gum tissue. In these cases, the teeth may be aligned with the transposed teeth remaining in the "incorrect" spots. After treatment, the teeth can be reshaped to look like the normal tooth in that spot. Other times, one of the transposed teeth can be extracted along with other teeth to treat the malocclusion.

Figure 19-11. Transposition of maxillary right lateral incisor and canine, before and after orthodontic treatment.

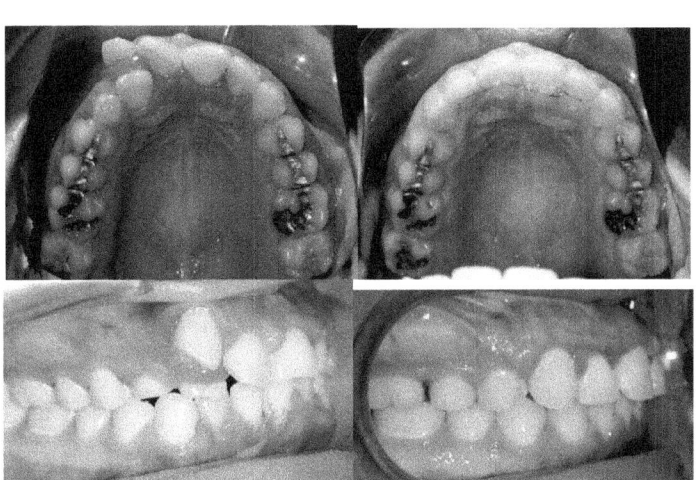

Missing Teeth

There are two kinds of missing teeth, and both introduce different nuances to orthodontic treatment plans.

Congenitally missing teeth are teeth that never developed and formed in your jaws. Instead of having 32 teeth develop, you would have fewer than 32. There may be a baby tooth in your mouth, and an x-ray would show no permanent tooth underneath the baby tooth. In children, you can sometimes extract the baby tooth and allow the back teeth to drift forward to close the extraction space. This would eliminate the need for a future restoration of the missing tooth. The baby tooth can be aligned and maintained with the other permanent teeth, if the roots aren't shrinking, if the tooth is healthy, and if the orthodontist thinks the tooth won't be lost in the near future. If the baby tooth has shrinking roots or big fillings, the orthodontist will want to extract the tooth. You can either replace the missing tooth with an implant or try to close the space with braces. The space left by the baby tooth is usually large and may be difficult to close orthodontically.

Adults may have had teeth extracted due to previous decay. Missing teeth can cause problems. The adjacent teeth tend to lean into the empty space. The opposing tooth that is supposed to chew against that missing tooth may continue to grow down into the empty space. So, periodontal problems can arise around adjacent teeth, tooth shifting can occur, and bites can change. Orthodontic treatment can upright the adjacent teeth to prepare for proper implant placement or bridge fabrication, in order to restore the empty space with a false tooth restoration. Sometimes the orthodontist can close the extraction space.

Peg Lateral Incisors

Teeth don't always come in the correct shape and size, and we already discussed how some teeth don't even develop at all. A common tooth to develop with the wrong shape is the maxillary lateral incisor, or the second tooth from the middle on the top arch. These teeth, fairly commonly, are skinnier than normal. They can be really thin and pointy, and these are referred to as "peg laterals."

No matter how straight your teeth are, a tooth with uncharacteristic anatomy can affect the fit of the teeth, or as in the case of the peg lateral, effect the look of the smile. Larger teeth can be slenderized (IPR) or smoothed down to a manageable shape. Peg laterals are too small and need to be built up. The orthodontist or general dentist can do this with a tooth colored filling material.

Your orthodontist will recommend building the tooth up either before, during, or after orthodontic treatment. Sometimes a peg lateral will have to be restored with a veneer or crown.

Temporary Anchorage Devices or Miniscrews

Some orthodontic movements are hard to accomplish. Closing large spaces or intruding molars are tough movements. Some of these tough movements can cause unwanted and negative effects on the other teeth. Temporary Anchorage Devices (TADs), or miniscrews, are useful tools to overcome the undesirable movements of the other teeth.

Every movement in orthodontics leads to an opposite reaction of the anchor teeth. For example, trying to close a large space by pulling the front teeth backwards causes the back to come forward. We want the back teeth to be anchors and not move, but inevitably they will move at least a little. To prevent movement of the teeth that we don't want to move, orthodontists can use the jaw bones for anchorage. TADs are tiny screws that are placed in the jaw bone. The orthodontic forces can be applied to the teeth we want to move, and anchored to the screws in the jaw instead of the teeth. The screw is stable and will not move. Examples of TAD treatments are shown in Figures 19-12, 19-13, 19-14, and 19-15.

Does this hurt? Placement of TADs is fairly easy and painless. The orthodontist will ensure that your gums are numb. He may use a topical anesthetic gel only, or he may decide to give an injection (shot). The screw is turned or screwed in the bone just like a wood screw. There is some pressure during insertion but no sharp or stinging pain. The screw site will feel sore maybe for 1 day. For removal, the orthodontist will apply the topical anesthetic gel and just unscrew the TAD. That is painless also.

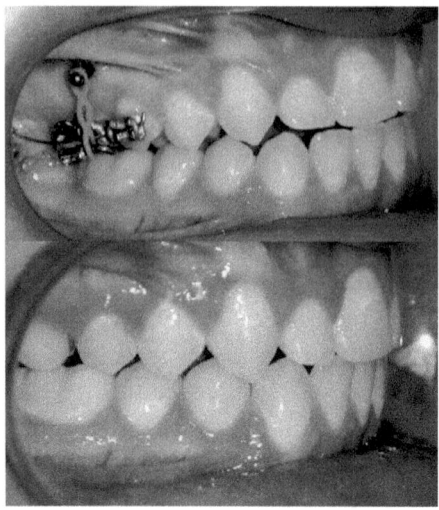

Figure 19-12. TAD used to intrude the maxillary molars and close the anterior openbite.

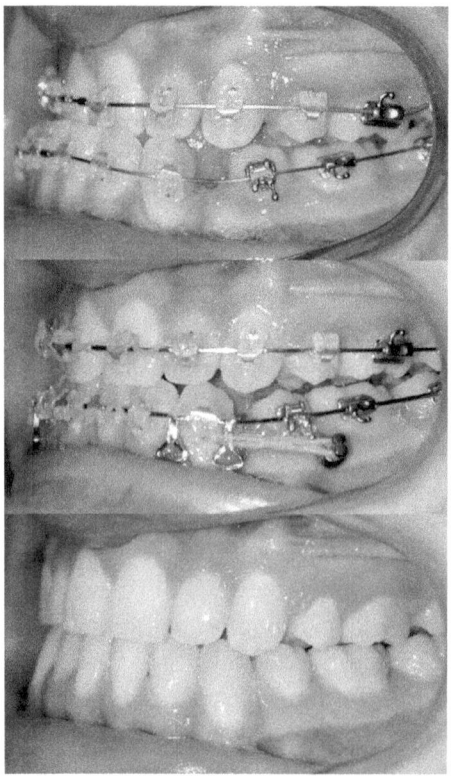

Figure 19-13. TAD used to close the lower extraction space by pulling the incisors back and preventing the molars from going forward.

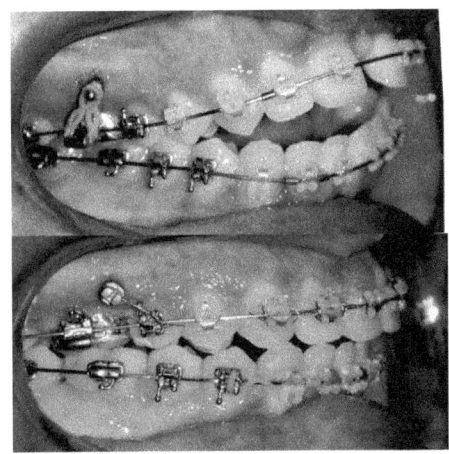

Figure 19-14.
TAD used to
intrude the maxillary
molars and close the
anterior openbite.

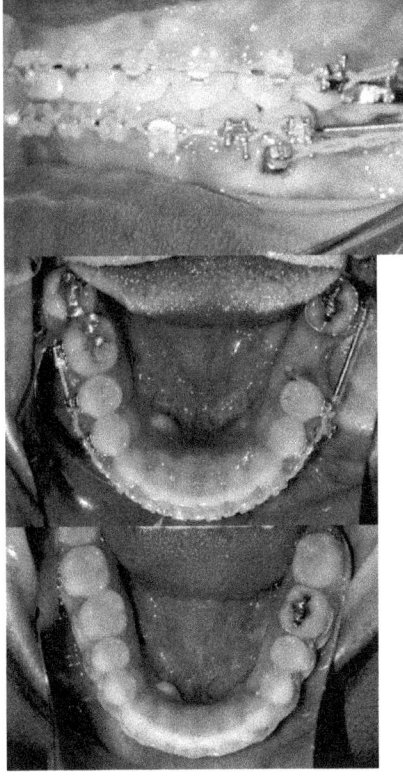

Figure 19-15.
TAD used to
pull the lower
molars
forward and
prevent the
anterior teeth
from moving
backward.

20

CLEANING AROUND BRACES AND TAKING CARE OF BRACES

It's the orthodontist's job to straighten your teeth, but it's your job to brush and clean your teeth. It's up to you to keep your entire mouth healthy so that your new beautiful smile will last a lifetime. Brushing and flossing your teeth regularly is essential to keep your mouth clean and healthy. Proper oral hygiene care with braces takes only a little extra effort and care.

Brushing and flossing

Plaque needs to be thoroughly removed from your teeth at least twice a day. When you have braces, it's even more important to remove plaque. All the brackets and wires in your mouth create places for plaque to hide. What is plaque? Plaque is a sticky mixture of food, saliva, and bacteria. This bacteria metabolizes foods and sugars to release acids that demineralize your teeth and cause decay. If plaque attaches to your braces and teeth, it can cause cavities, swollen gums, bad breath, and permanent stain marks on your teeth.

If possible, you should brush your teeth after every time you eat. If you can't actually brush with a toothbrush, then at least rinse your mouth out with water. This will loosen and remove some of the food from your braces. Travel toothbrushes are easy to carry and very useful.

Brushing twice a day is important, but you should also clean between your teeth with floss at least once every day. Floss first, and then brush your teeth and braces thoroughly until they're clean. The best time to do this thorough cleaning is at night, right before you go to bed.

You still need to see your dentist every 6 months (or more frequently if your orthodontist recommends) for regular checkups. Your dentist and hygienist will make sure your mouth and teeth are clean, and they can also address any questions you have regarding brushes, floss, other oral hygiene aids, and tips for cleaning braces in any area of your mouth that you find difficult to reach.

Brushing your teeth when you have braces isn't that much different than brushing your teeth without braces. You should use a soft bristle toothbrush or power toothbrush, and brush for a full two minutes. You should replace your toothbrush about every 3 months, because the bristles of the toothbrush will wear out faster when brushing against the braces. You should brush around all the parts of your teeth, including the fronts, sides, backs, and chewing surfaces, along with your tongue and roof of your mouth. Angle the toothbrush so that it scrubs the top and bottom of the braces.

Your dentist or orthodontist may prescribe fluoride toothpaste or gel to help you fight tooth decay even more. Brush gently but thoroughly. Brush carefully, not harder. If your braces look clean and shiny and if you can see the edges of the brackets clearly, you've done a good job! Make sure to rinse your mouth after brushing. Mouth rinses may be beneficial.

Yes, flossing is a challenge. It takes a little more time flossing around the archwires and braces. It can be done! Remember to carefully go under the gum line. A floss threader may help. A floss threader is a tool that allows dental floss to get underneath the archwires easily. There are a lot of other hygiene aids that might be even easier for you to use.

The braces will not damage your teeth, but poor oral hygiene and plaque around the braces can damage your teeth. As long as you maintain good oral habits, you don't have to worry about cavities and decay around the braces. Brushing, flossing, and seeing your dentist for a cleaning every six months will prevent problems associated with poor oral hygiene. Poor oral hygiene problems affect people whether they have braces or not. When people have braces some problems can be worse if you don't brush and floss like you should.

Gingivitis, or gum disease, is inflammation of the gum tissue. It is the first stage of periodontal disease. It's usually painless. There may be some bleeding or swollen gums. This happens when plaque builds up around the gum line, so make sure to massage your gums lightly when you brush, as well as floss well along the gum line.

Periodontitis results from untreated and prolonged gingivitis. Inflammation in the gums spreads deeper to the bone that supports the teeth. The gums start to pull away, forming gaps or pockets between your teeth that allow more plaque to accumulate.

Decalcifications or "white spots" are permanent stains around your braces. They result, not from the braces, but from plaque that accumulates around the braces. Decalcification spots and lines stay on your teeth for life, so preventing them is really important. Brushing and flossing properly will prevent these spots. If they are severe, your dentist may have to drill out the decalcification and restore with a filling. It should be noted that soft drinks and sports drinks accelerate the decalcification process, so you should limit these or avoid these when you have braces.

What foods should I avoid when wearing braces?

Braces are strong and stable, but you need to treat these orthodontic appliances with care. The braces will stay in place when you eat foods that are gentle on the brackets and wires. Try to avoid all foods that are sticky, hard, or chewy. Soft foods are recommended for those who wear braces because they are simply easier on your mouth, jaws, and appliances. Again, try to stay away from soft drinks and sports drinks.

Foods to avoid when bearing braces:
- Popcorn
- Nuts
- Hard taco shells
- Sticky and hard candy
- Gum
- Ice
- Crunchy chips
- Pretzels
- Hard cookies or crackers
- Sticky or hard chocolate

Also avoid biting into hard foods with your front teeth. Cut or break up hard foods such as:

- Raw vegetables
- French/Italian bread
- Fruit
- Hard rolls
- Thin crust pizza
- Meat
- Burgers
- Sub sandwiches
- Corn on the cob

21

ORTHOGNATHIC SURGERY

Sometimes the misalignment of the teeth isn't just a matter of crooked teeth. There can also be underlying jaw discrepancies that contribute to a bad bite. Often, these abnormalities cause difficulty associated with everyday functions like chewing, talking, sleeping and other routine activities. To fix a bite like this would take more than just braces and orthodontics. Corrective jaw surgery (orthognathic surgery) treats and corrects abnormalities of the facial bones, specifically the jaws and the teeth. Orthognathic surgery corrects these problems and, in conjunction with orthodontic treatment, will improve the overall appearance of the facial profile.

The orthodontist or oral surgeon will demonstrate the overall functional and esthetic benefits of orthognathic surgery should you need it. Computerized treatment planning realistically predicts treatment times, treatment outcomes, and recovery periods, improving the overall efficacy of your surgery. State-of-the-art materials such as titanium plates and miniature screws provide stability, strength, and predictability to your treatment. These advances in technology, procedures, and equipment reduce post-surgical recovery time, thus allowing patients to return to their normal routines soon after the surgery.

Orthognathic surgeries aren't done until the patient is completely done growing. The earliest age oral surgeons will do surgeries is 16 for girls and 16 or 17 in boys. Surgeries can be done at any stage of adulthood. Typically, braces are put on before the surgery. Initial alignment is done for about a year. The surgery will be done after the tooth alignment and while the braces are still there. The patient will then finish the orthodontic treatment, and the braces can be removed about 6 months after the surgery.

Surgeries can be used to move one or both of the jaws in any direction. Common examples include moving the mandible forward, the maxilla forward, the mandible backward, the maxilla upward, or the mandible asymmetrically (backward more on one side).

It is becoming more difficult to find insurances that cover the cost of orthognathic surgeries. Your oral surgeon can help you discover if any coverage exists with your plan.

Orthognathic surgery may be unnecessary if orthodontic treatment can correct the problem. With the latest advances in orthodontics, this is sometimes the case.

Does this hurt? Most people report the same discomfort as wisdom tooth removal. There is some tenderness, swelling, and inability to open fully for a couple of weeks after the surgery. If two jaws undergo operation, then the pain and discomfort may last a little longer. Single-jaw surgeries are sometimes done as outpatient procedures with no overnight hospital stay. You may have to stay in the hospital a couple of nights if both jaws undergo surgery. While the bones of your jaws heal, the surgeon may ask you to avoid sports for 6 weeks.

22

HOW DOES THE ORTHODONTIST TAKE THE BRACES OFF MY TEETH?

Removing braces from the teeth is a simple procedure. Special debonding pliers are made for this event. The pliers are placed around the bracket, and with a simple squeeze, the bracket is separated from the tooth. You may hear a click or snap as the adhesive breaks to free the bracket.

Ceramic brackets are removed the same way. Sometimes the orthodontist drills off a little of the extra adhesive first. Then he will use some pliers to grab the bracket. With a little squeeze, the bracket pops off the tooth. There is a louder snapping sound with ceramic brackets, and maybe a little more pressure with the squeeze. Occasionally, the ceramic brackets crack, and the orthodontist will simply grind off the remaining piece of bracket with a handpiece (drill).

To remove bands, the orthodontist uses a debanding plier. He grabs the band and uses pressure against the tooth. Again, a loud sound may be heard as the cement holding the band in place will break to release the band.

Then the band slides off the tooth.

After the brackets are off the teeth, a square shaped patch of adhesive will remain on the teeth. The orthodontist will remove this with a dental handpiece that shaves the adhesive away or a plier that scratches off the adhesive. The cement left over from a band will most likely be removed with a handpiece.

Does this hurt? Removing the braces does not hurt. A small pressure may be felt when the orthodontist handles the pliers. Occasionally, one tooth may be sensitive, and the orthodontist will have an answer for that. The ceramic brackets require a little extra force, but it is easily tolerated and not painful. The bands come off with a loud snap, but that is painless. Removing the glue is also painless.

23

RETAINERS

Now your braces are off. Your teeth are straight and your smile is beautiful! Unfortunately, teeth have a tendency to move back to the crooked positions. There is a tendency for relapse. Even though the teeth probably will not return to the exact position where they were before orthodontic treatment, it can be frustrating and sad when your new beautiful smile starts to change. You worked for that smile; you wore braces for almost 2 years! Retainers prevent the teeth from relapsing.

Retainers come in many different designs. There are removable retainers and bonded (fixed or permanent) retainers. They are custom made for your teeth, and the type of retainer you should have is determined by your initial malocclusion.

Removable retainers (Figure 22-1) are most commonly made from acrylic and a metal wire. The acrylic fits along the lingual surfaces of your teeth and the palate (for a upper retainer). The metal is referred to as a bow, and it fits along the buccal surfaces of your teeth. The bow can be adjusted to slightly move teeth in some cases. Special hooks and springs can be added to move teeth or control their new positions. Clasps can be added to make the retainer fit snugly on the teeth. These retainers are durable and long lasting. You can clean these by brushing with a toothbrush and rinsing with cool or warm (not hot) water.

Another removable retainer is the clear aligner (Figure 13-1). These may discolor over time and probably have to be replaced in the future. You can clean these by running them under cool or warm water (not hot) and brushing with a toothbrush.

Removable retainers should be worn for the time recommended by the orthodontist. At a minimum, they should be worn during bedtime, every night. You may be advised to wear them during the day right after your braces are removed. If you skip nights or take breaks from wearing these, your teeth may shift and move!

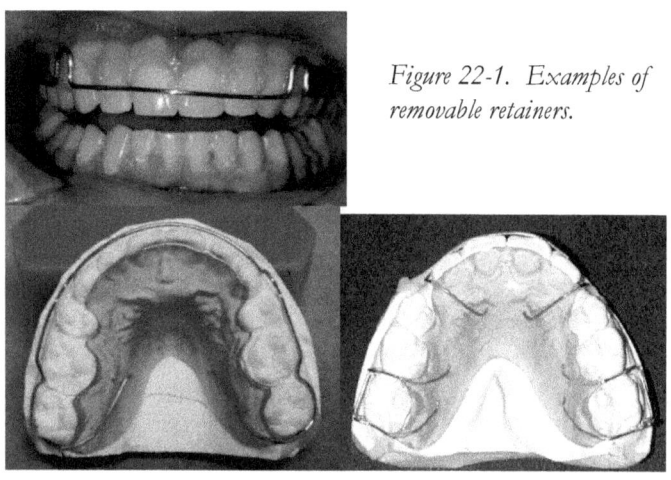

Figure 22-1. Examples of removable retainers.

Bonded or fixed retainers (Figure 22-2) overcome the need to depend on patients to faithfully wear removable retainers. A wire is adapted to the lingual surfaces of the teeth, and orthodontic adhesive is used to glue the retainers in place. Bonded retainers are common for lower incisors, as these are the teeth most likely to relapse. Depending on your bite, upper bonded retainers are more difficult to place without your lower teeth hitting it when you chew. Upper bonded retainers are more likely to break and need repairs. Bonded retainers are difficult to floss around, and they may hold on to more plaque. Your orthodontist will determine how long you wear a bonded retainer, but these can usually stay in place indefinitely.

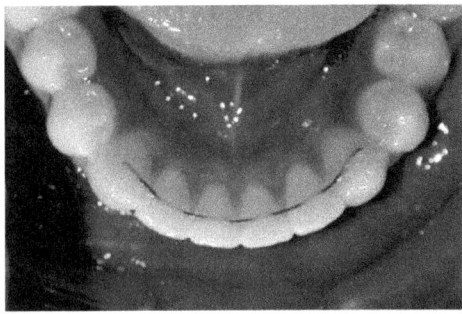

Figure 22-2. Fixed, bonded retainer on the lower incisors.

Patients who have TMJ problems or TMD may need a splint or nightguard (Figure 22-3) to make their jaws comfortable. Splints are used to stabilize the bite and are slightly more bulky than retainers. They can be made to fit the upper or lower teeth, and they do a pretty good job as retainers.

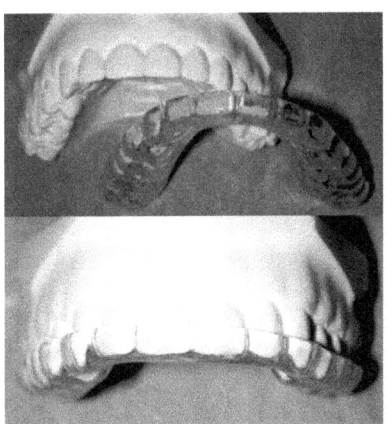

Figure 22-3. Splint for TMD patients, off and on the teeth.

Here are some tips for wearing your retainers:

- Wear your retainers full time, or as the doctor instructed.
- Take your retainers out when eating…and always put retainers in their case! (Most appliances are lost in school lunchrooms or restaurants).
- Clean retainers thoroughly once a day with a toothbrush and toothpaste. Use warm but not hot water. Brushing retainers removes the plaque, and eliminates odors. Denture cleaner or other orthodontic appliance cleaners can be used, but do not take the place of brushing.
- When retainers are not in your mouth they should ALWAYS be in a retainer case. Pets love to chew on them!
- Initially, you may find it difficult to speak while wearing retainers. Practice speaking, reading, or singing out loud to get used to them faster.
- Retainers are breakable, so treat them with care. If retainers are lost or broken call the orthodontist immediately.
- If you have any questions or concerns about your retainers, or if your retainers need adjusting, call the orthodontist. Do not try to adjust them yourself!
- Always bring your retainers to your appointments.
- Retainer replacement is expensive…with proper care they will last for years!
- Remove retainers when swimming.
- Keep retainers away from hot water, hot car dashboards, pockets, the washing machine, and napkins.

24

WHAT IS TMJ or TMD?

Pain or popping of the jaw bones is sometimes referred to as "TMJ" or "TMD." The temperomandibular joint is the connection of the mandible to the head. There is a disc that separates the two bones. The abbreviation for this joint is "TMJ." "TMD" is an abbreviation for temperomandibular joint disorders. So, pain associated with the temperomandibular joint or the muscles around the joint is correctly called TMD instead of TMJ.

There are many factors associated with pain of the TMJ. Occlusal instability or teeth that don't fit together correctly is a small factor. Physical irregularities of the joint can cause pain and clicking. Osteoarthritis can cause breakdown of the joint and pain. The most important factor and most common predisposing factor of TMJ pain is emotional stress. Anything in life that causes anxiety or stress can lead to changes in muscle activity and clenching, causing pain. Commonly, TMD starts in patients who clench and grind their teeth at night during their sleep. This bruxism is a subconscious habit that isn't under your direct control. Clenching and grinding overworks and fatigues the muscles of the TMJ, leading to pain. This pain can be felt around the masseter muscles along the sides of your lower jaw in front of your ears or around the temporal areas of your head above your ears. One way to control this nighttime clenching is to use a splint or nightguard (Figure 22-3).

Children, divorce, change in jobs, stressful occupations, holidays, or anything that weighs on your mind is considered a source of emotional stress. Everyone reacts to and handles stress differently.

Some people can feel or hear a clicking sound when they open and close their mouths. The clicking can become louder, and it is described as a pop. Sometimes, the jaw can lock in an open position or closed position. These noises of the TMJ are part of a progression of joint deterioration. The ligaments that hold the joint together and ensure proper function begin to loosen. Once the ligaments loosen, the disc that sits between the mandibular condyle and the glenoid fossa begins to slip forward and away from the stable position. The slipping of the disc out of the joint space is felt as a click or pop. When the disc fully leaves the joint space and prevents the mandible from freely moving, this is felt as a lock. Clicking or popping can also be the result of physical irregularities of the bones too, like bone spurs.

About half the population can feel a click on one side of their heads. A click alone is not TMD. A disorder is recognized as pain intensifies, clicking becomes really frequent, and function of the jaws becomes limited. Treatment of TMD can range from modifying lifestyles to splints and orthodontic treatment. Lifestyle changes include stopping gum-chewing (which overworks the muscles of mastication), softer diets, smaller bites, and posture changes. Massaging the jaws and stretching the muscles periodically can help. Splints that stabilize the bite or specifically posture the mandible may be indicated. Orthodontic treatment may also be recommended to fix the bite and stabilize the occlusion. Your orthodontist may even prescribe medications ranging from ibuprofen to muscle relaxers or antidepressant medications.

Appendix: Examples of Comprehensive Treatment,Before and After Photos

App 1A and 1B. Non-extraction treatment. Class I, deep bite, mild crowding, excessive gingival display in smile, and narrow arches.

App 1A

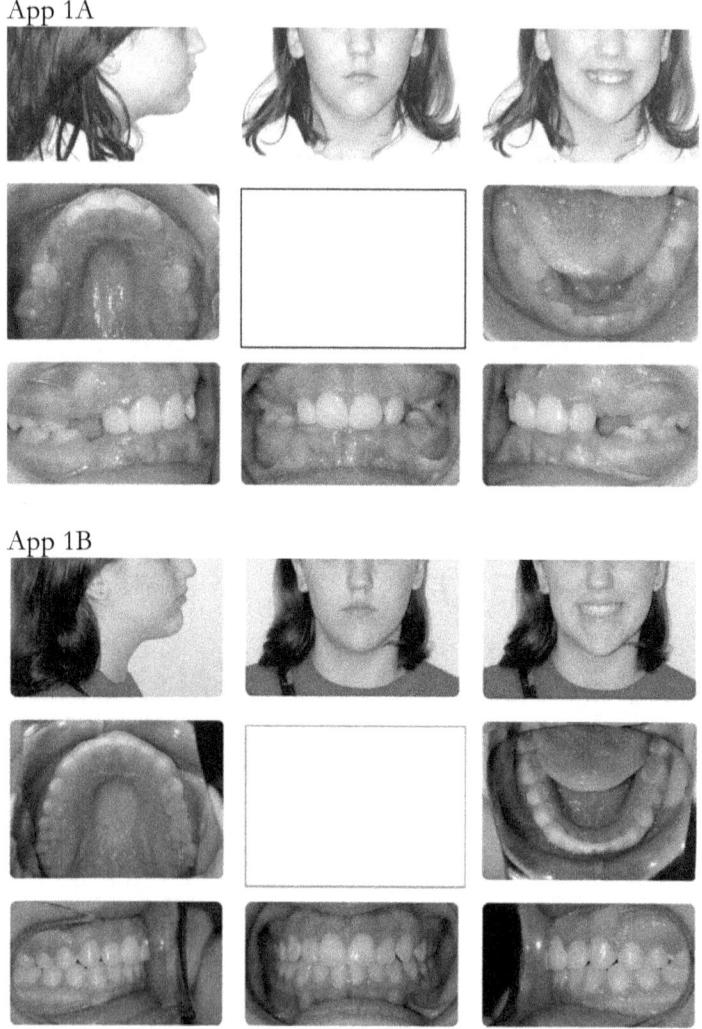

App 1B

App 2A and 2B. Non-extraction treatment. Class I, upper spacing, lower crowding, small maxillary lateral incisors, protrusive maxillary incisors, and open bite. The maxillary lateral incisors were built-up after orthodontic treatment.

App 2A

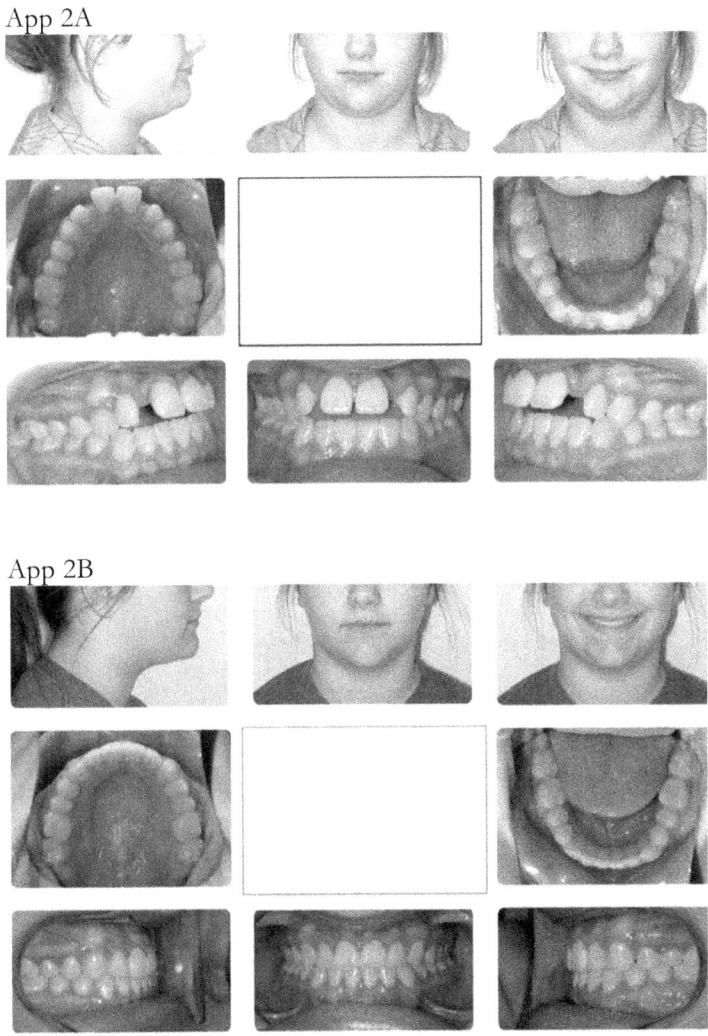

App 2B

App 3A and 3B. Non-extraction treatment. Class II, deep bite, upper crowding, lower spacing, and lower midline off to the left. Class II correcting springs were used.

App 3A

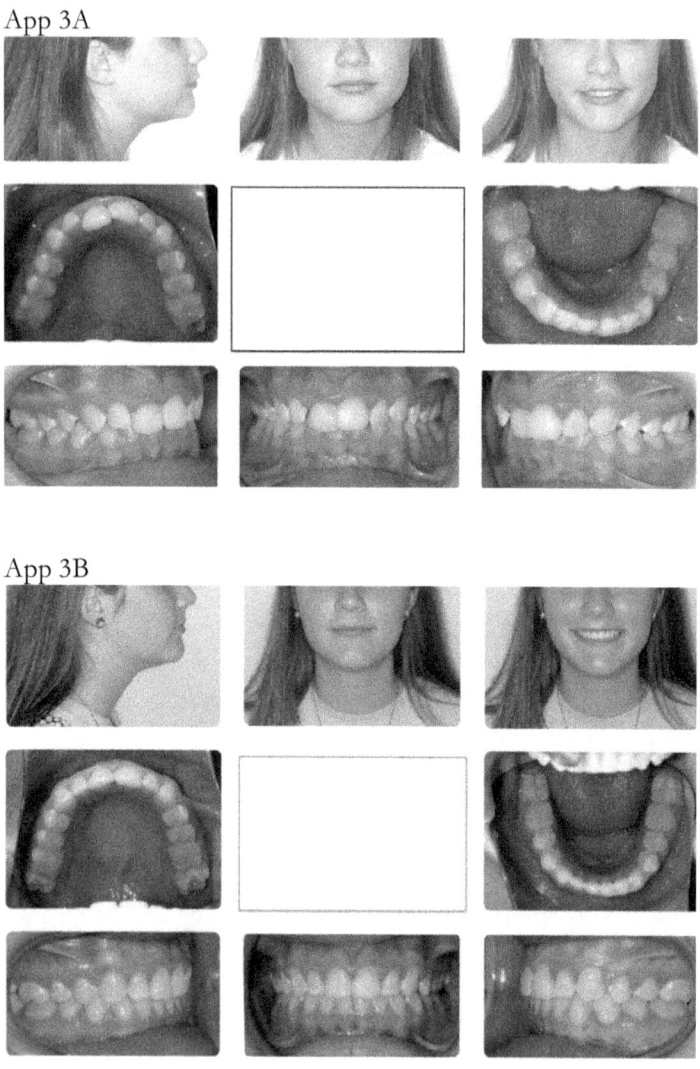

App 4A and 4B. Extraction of 4 premolars. Class I, moderate crowding, upper midline off to the left, lower midline off to the right, and blocked out maxillary left canine.

App 4A

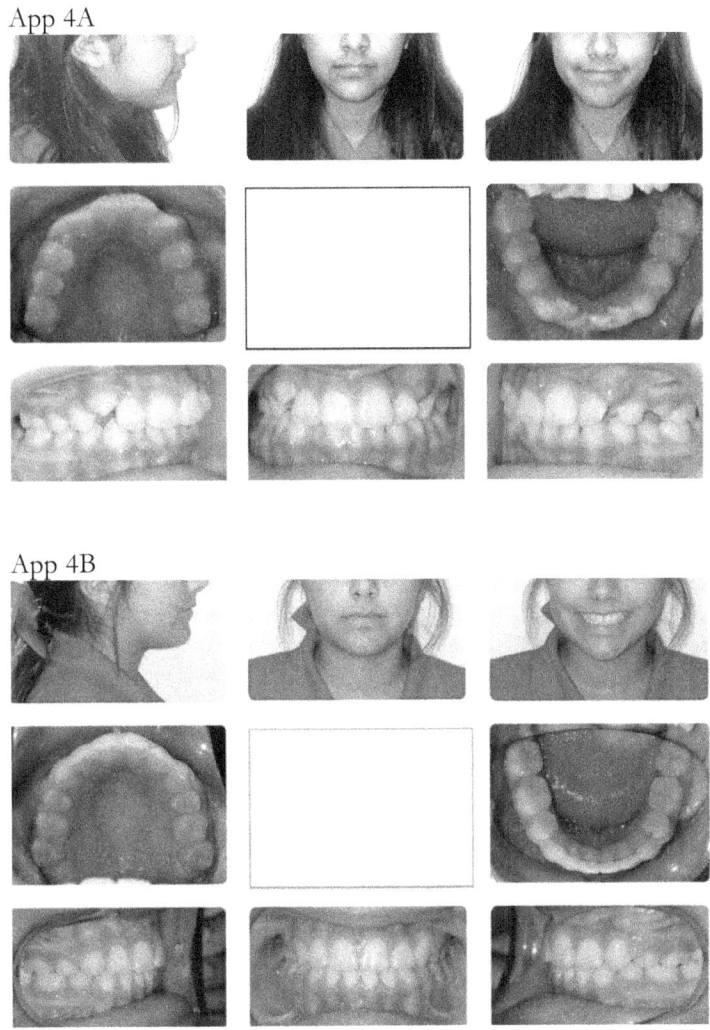

App 4B

App 5A and 5B. Extraction of 3 premolars (2 upper and one lower). Class II, moderate crowding, posterior crossbite, deep bite, narrow upper arch, and lower midline off to the left.

App 5A

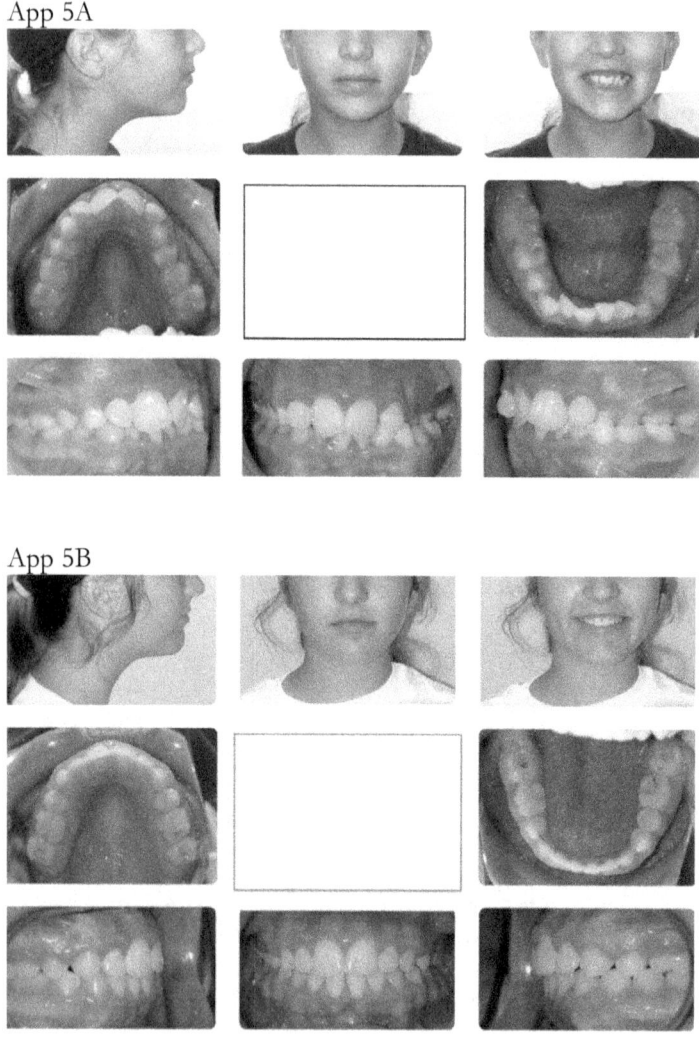

App 5B

App 6A and 6B. Non-extraction treatment. Class II, mild crowding, deep bite, and retroclined maxillary incisors. Class II correcting springs were used.

App 6A

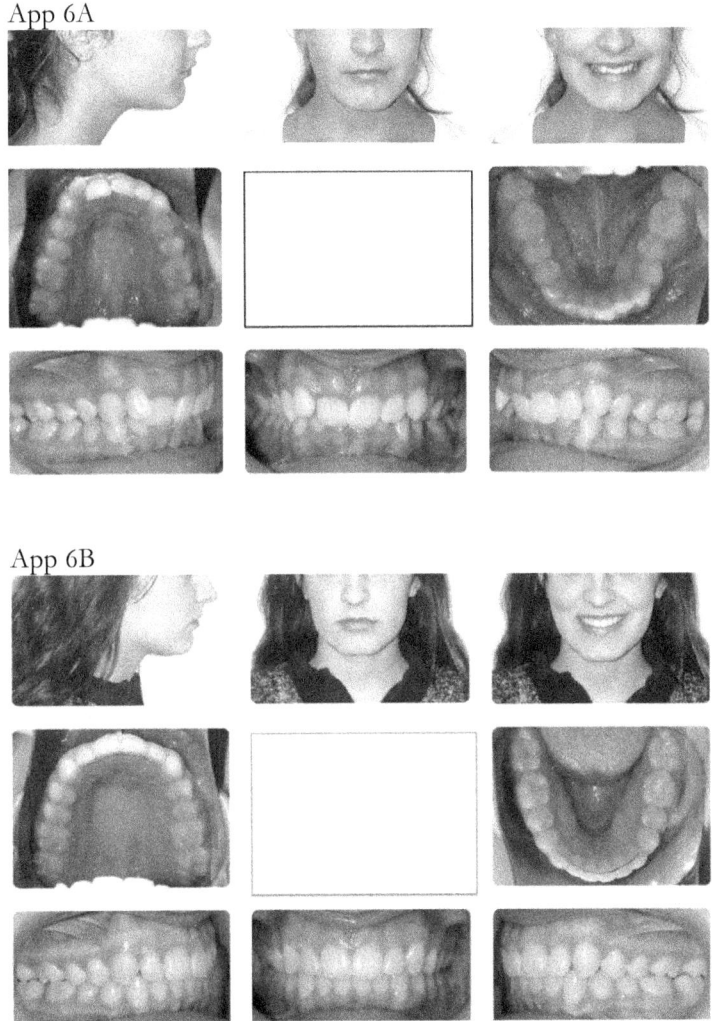

App 7A and 7B. Non-extraction treatment. Class I, open bite, over-retained maxillary right primary canine, moderate spacing, and upper midline off to the left.

App 7A

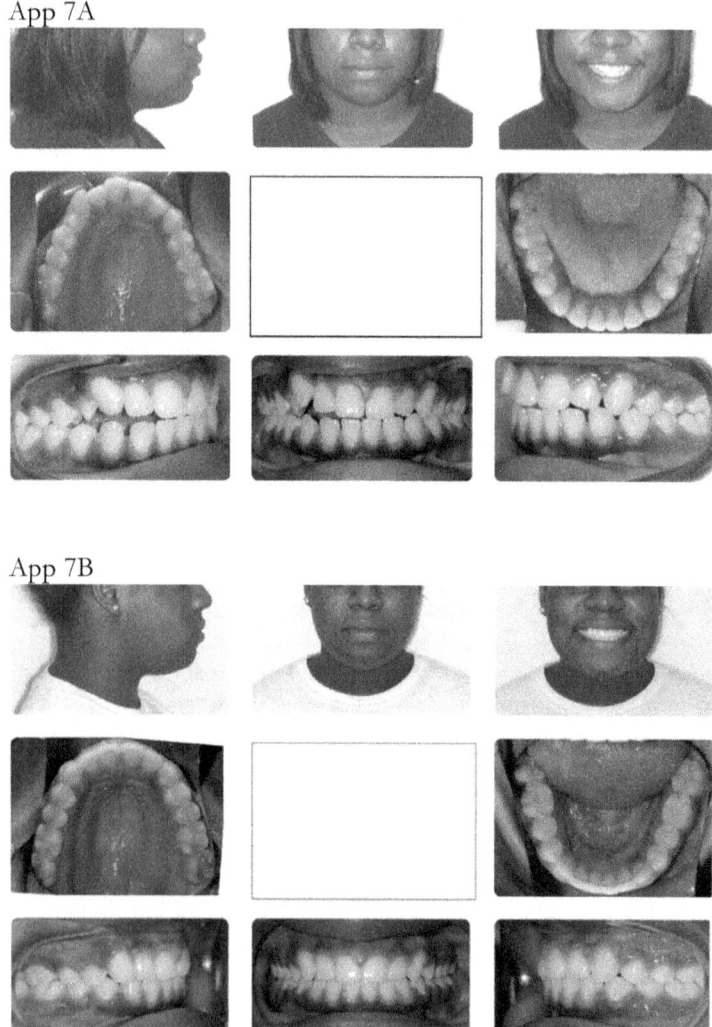

App 7B

App 8A and 8B. Non-extraction treatment. Class III, forward functional shift of the mandible, underbite, deep bite, upper crowding, and lower spacing.

App 8A

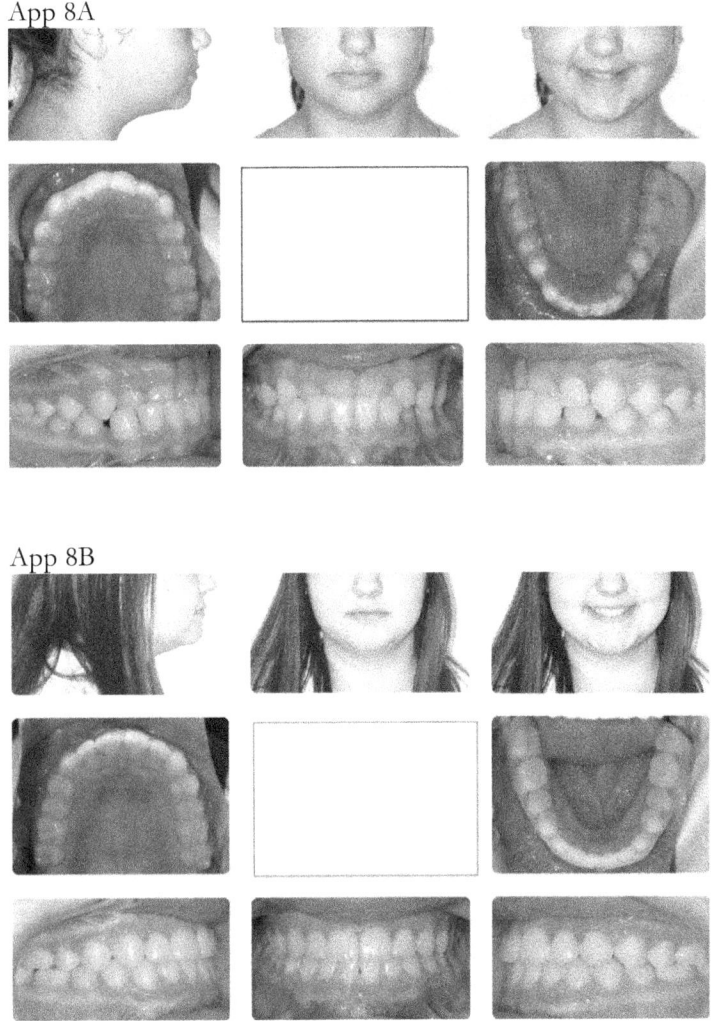

App 8B

App 9A and 9B. Non-extraction treatment. Class I, posterior crossbite, anterior crossbite, functional shift of the mandible, narrow upper arch, and mild crowding.

App 9A

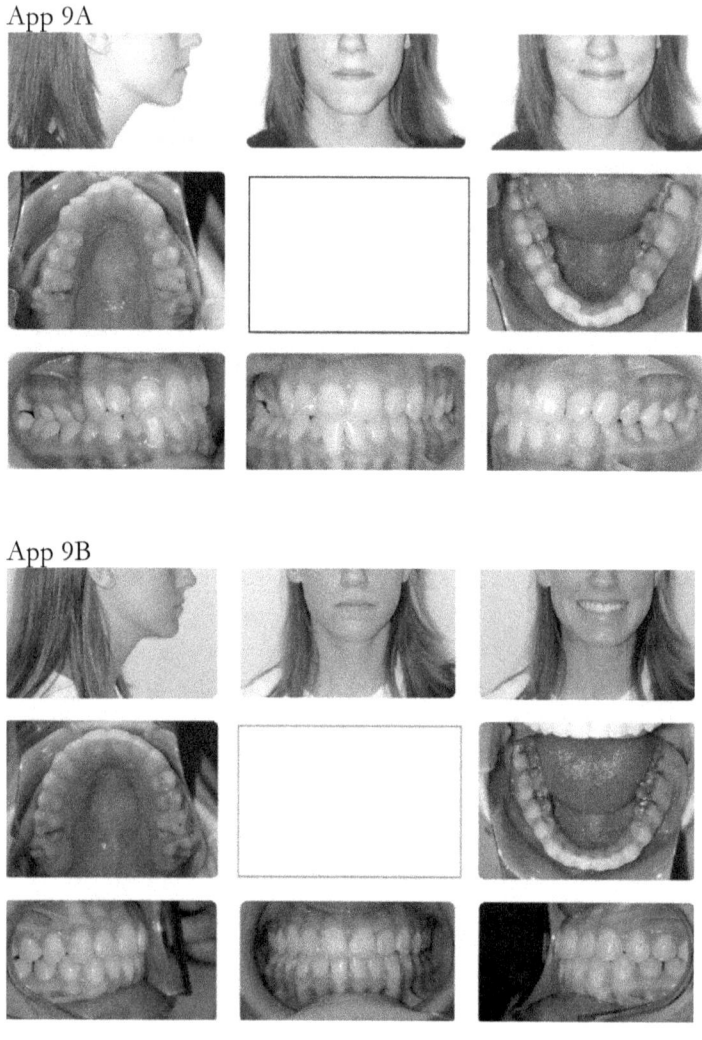

App 9B

App 10A and 10B. Extraction of 4 premolars. Class III, moderate crowding, open bite tendency, lower midline off to the right, blocked out maxillary left canine, and blocked out mandibular right canine.

App 10A

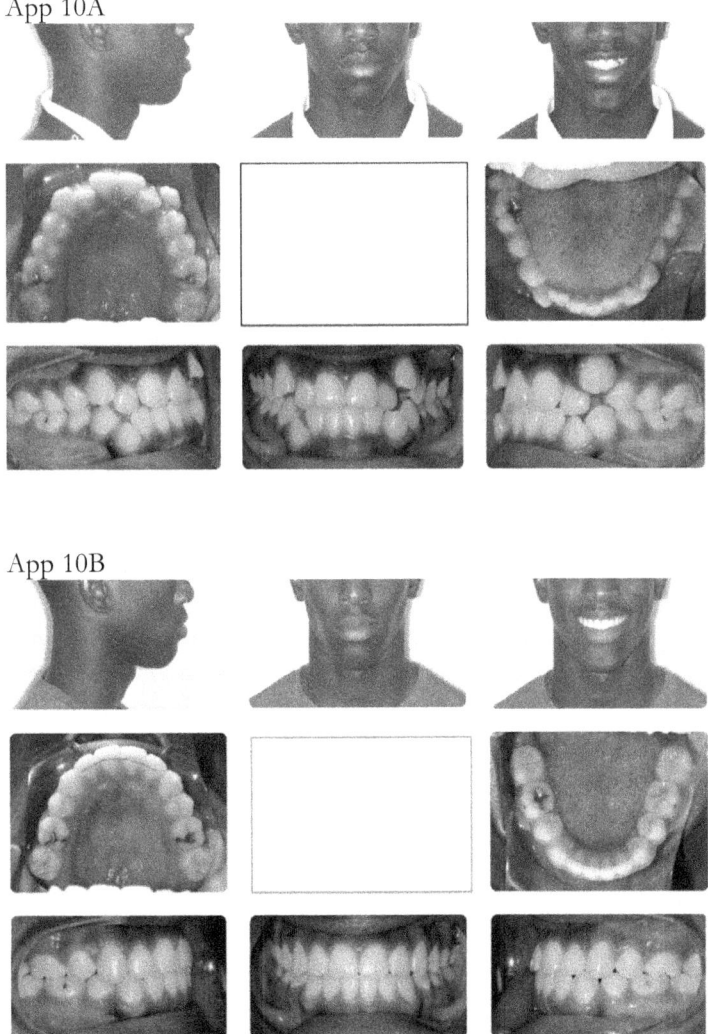

App 10B

App 11A and 11B. Extraction of 4 premolars. Class I, moderate crowding, protrusive upper and lower incisors, mandibular midline off to the left, mild lip strain, and protrusive lip profile.

App 11A

App 11B

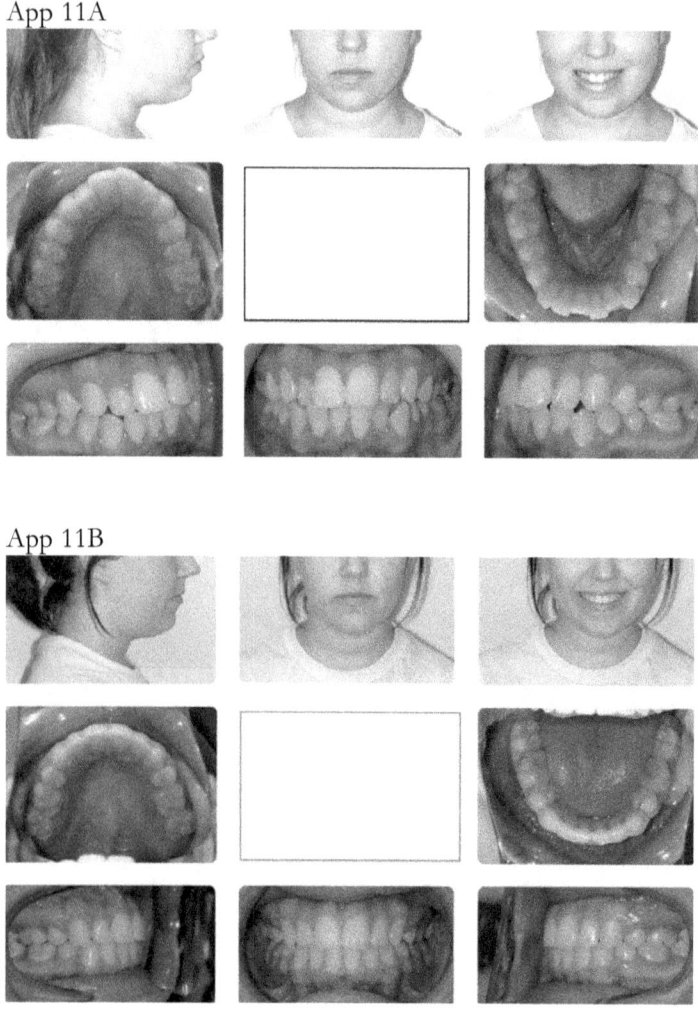

App 12A and 12B. Non-extraction treatment.
Class I, anterior crossbite, and moderate crowding.

App 12A

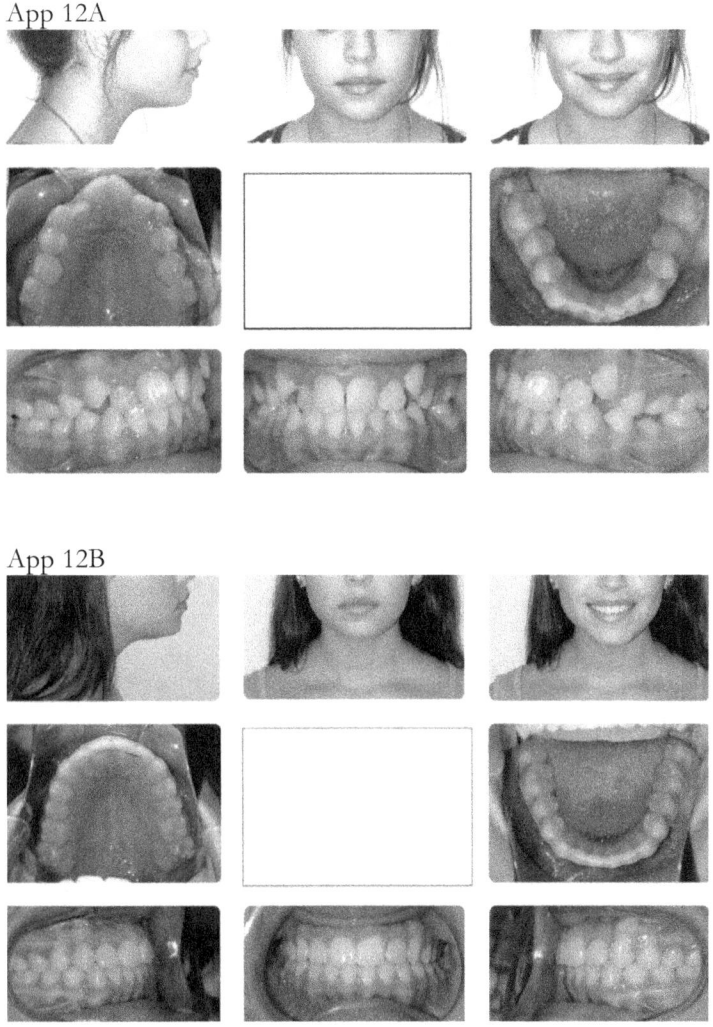

App 12B

App 13A and 13B. Non-extraction treatment. Class I, protrusive upper incisors, maxillary midline diastema, anterior open bite, and lower spacing.

App 13A

App 13B

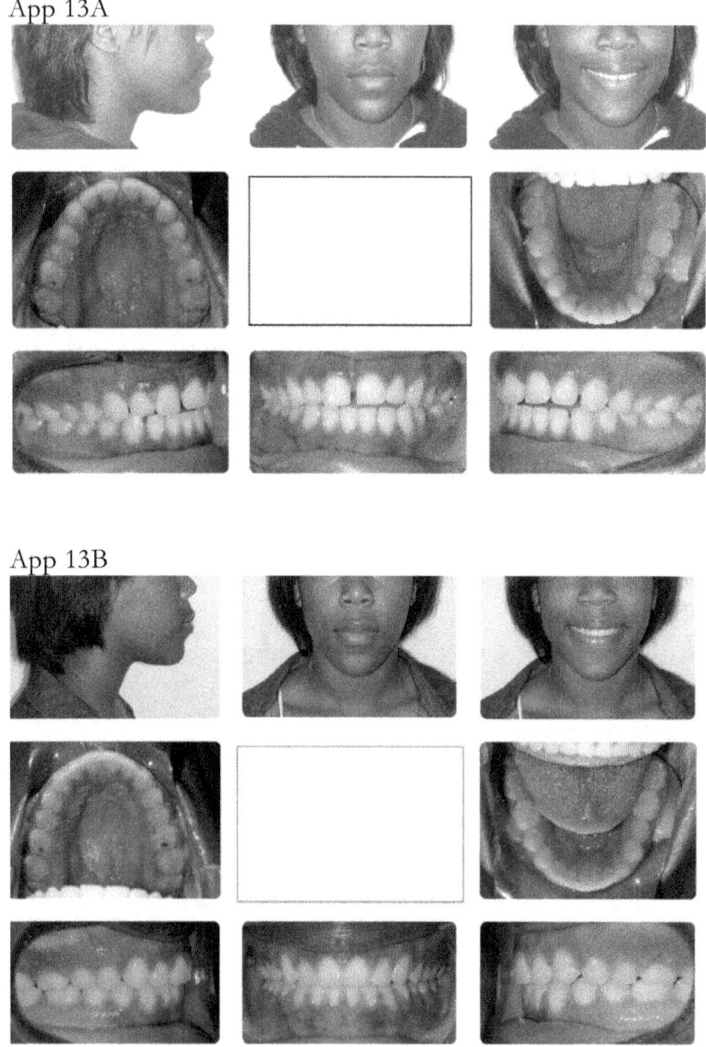

App 14A and 14B. Non-extraction treatment.
Class I, congenitally missing maxillary right lateral incisor,
peg maxillary left lateral incisor, and congenitally missing
left second molars (upper and lower). The space for the
missing maxillary right incisor was closed, and the
posterior teeth were shifted forward. The peg lateral
incisor on the right was restored to a normal shape and
size.

App 14A

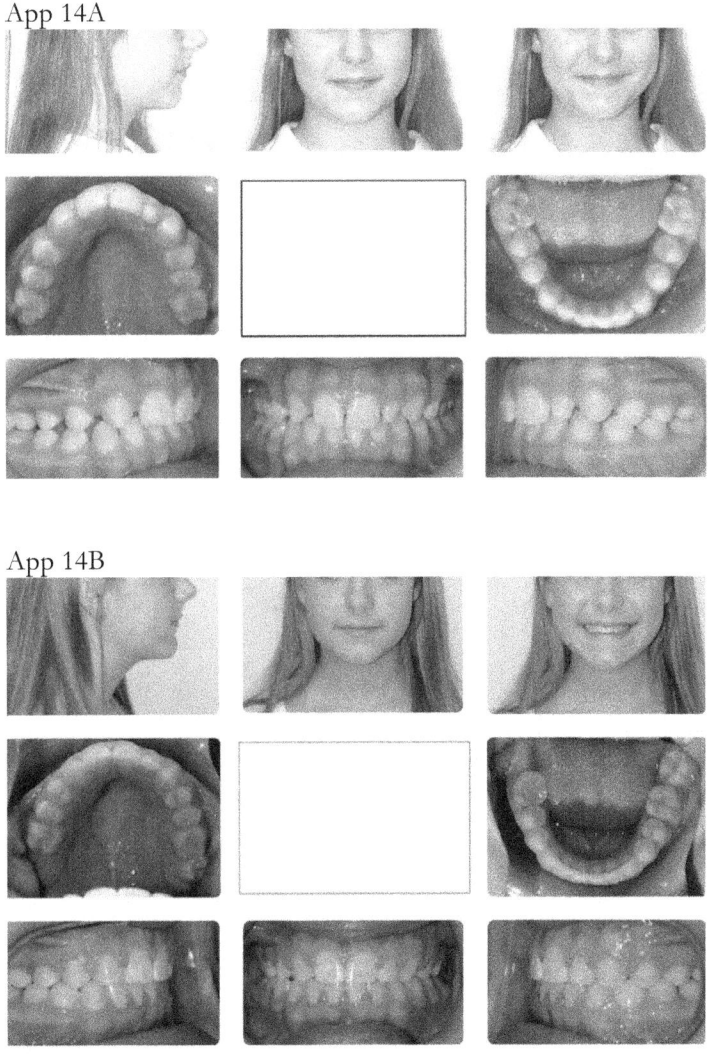

App 14B

App 15A and 15B. Extraction of 1 lower premolar. Class III, lateral open bite, mild lower crowding, anterior crossbite, and lower midline off to the left (due to an asymmetric mandible).

App 15A

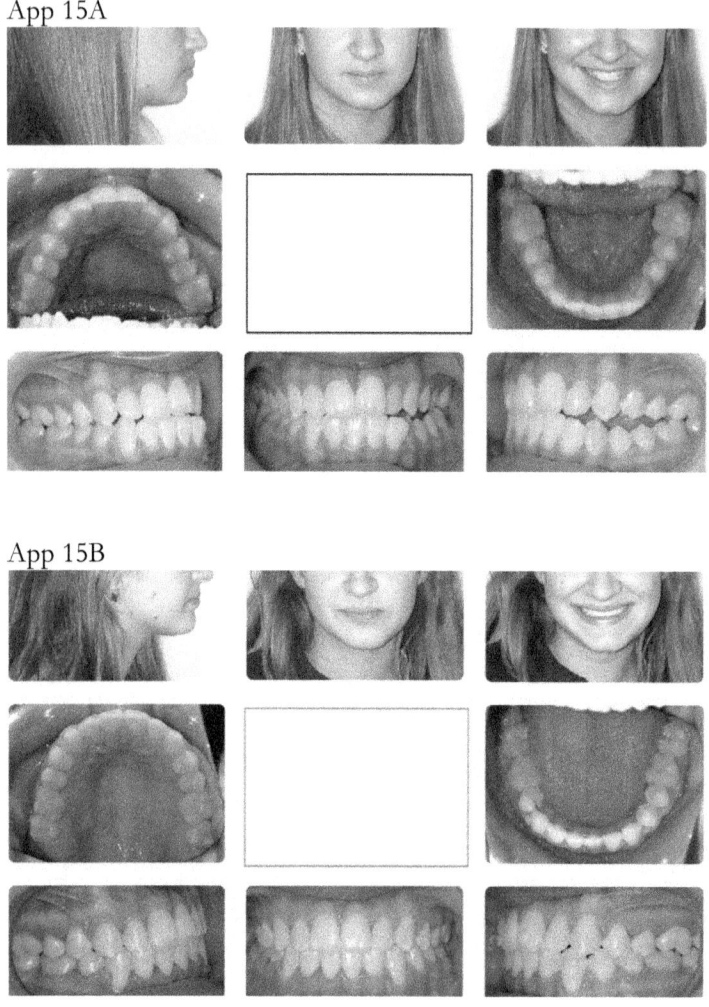

App 15B

App 16A and 16B. Non-extraction treatment. Class I, moderate crowding, and bilateral posterior crossbites.

App 16A

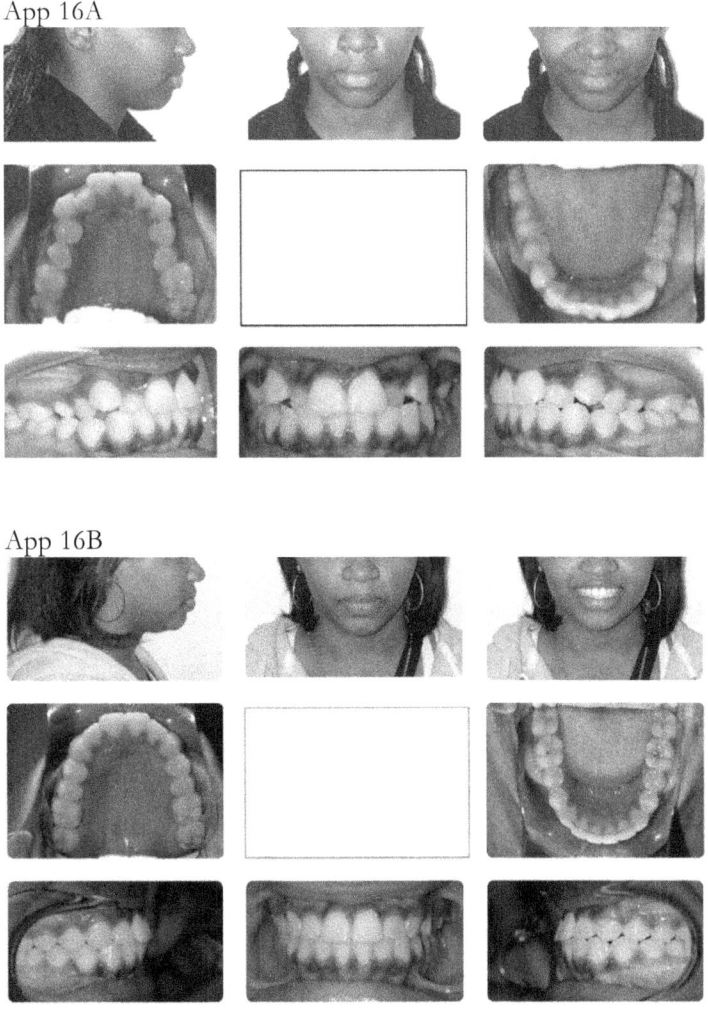

App 16B

App 17A and 17B. Extraction of 4 premolars. Class I, protrusive upper and lower incisors, mild lip strain, mild crowding, open bite tendency, and lower midline off to the left.

App 17A

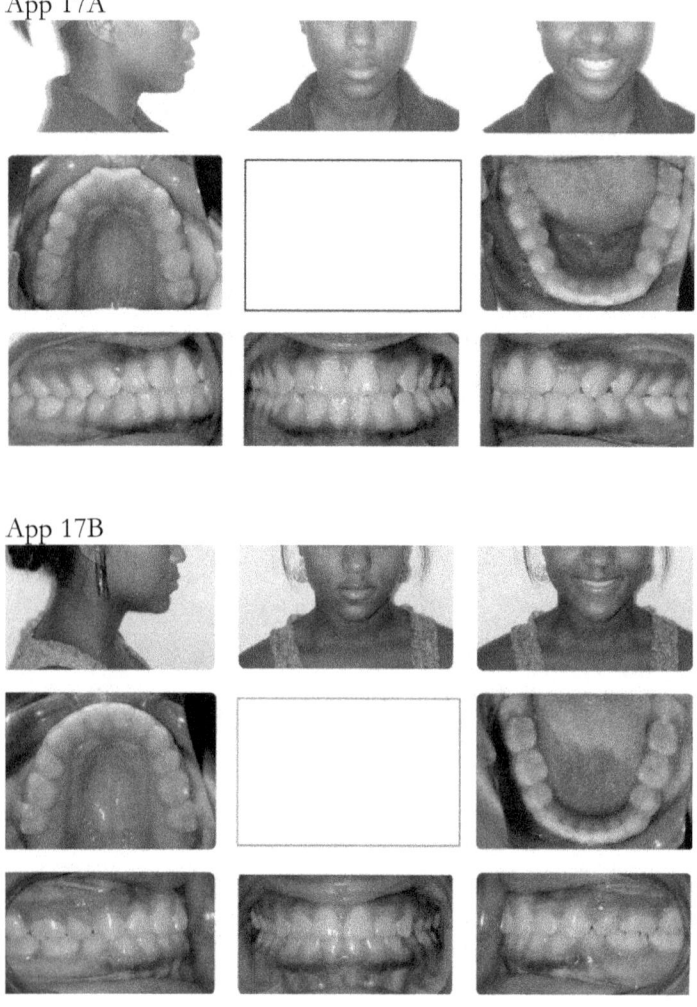

App 17B

App 18A and 18B. Extraction of 2 upper premolars. Class II, protrusive upper and lower incisors, excess overjet, deep bite, protrusive upper lip, and mild upper crowding.

App 18A

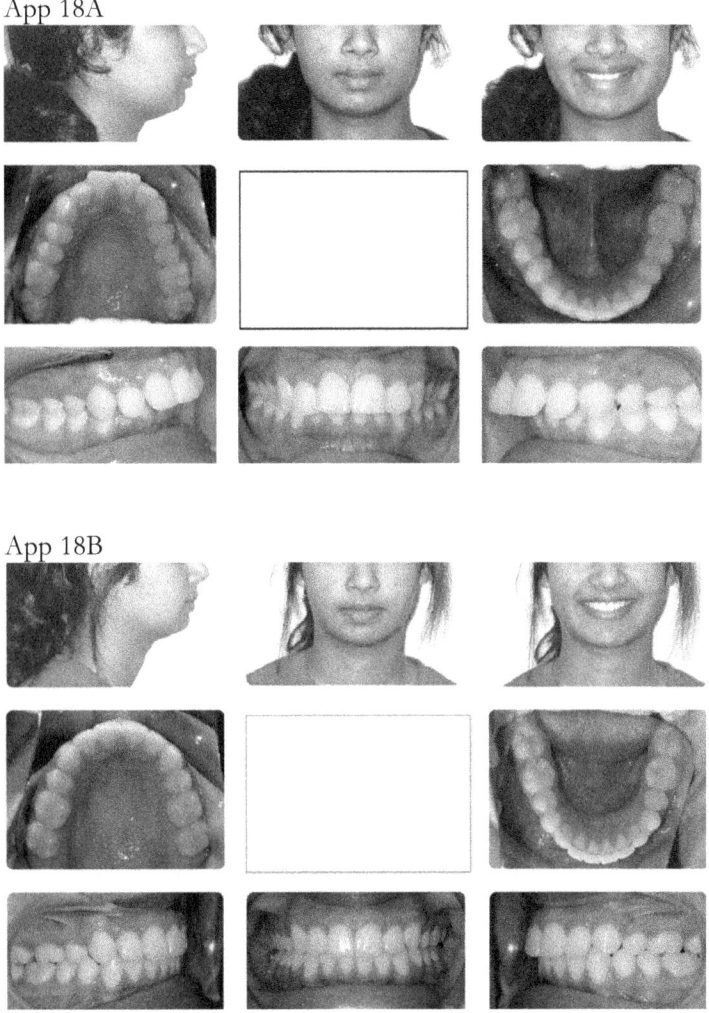

App 18B

App 19A and 19B. Non-extraction treatment. Class I, posterior crossbite, narrow upper arch, and moderate lower crowding. A rapid maxillary expander was used.

App 19A

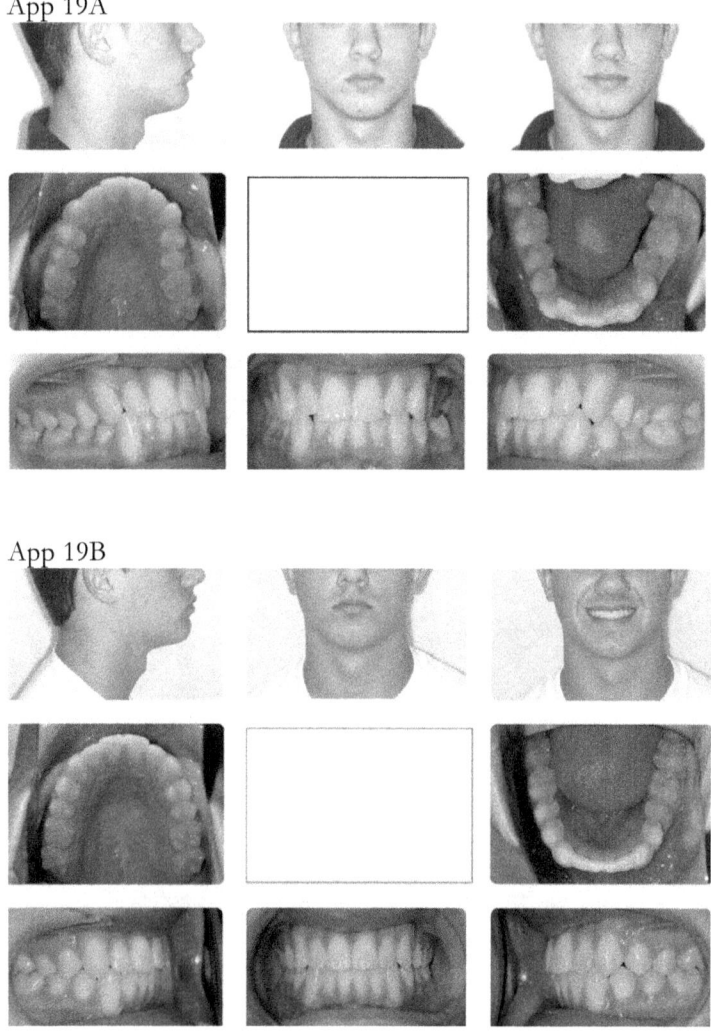

App 19B

App 20A and 20B. Non-extraction treatment.
Class II, deep bite, mild crowding, and retroclined and
over-erupted maxillary central incisors. Class II
correcting springs were used.

App 20A

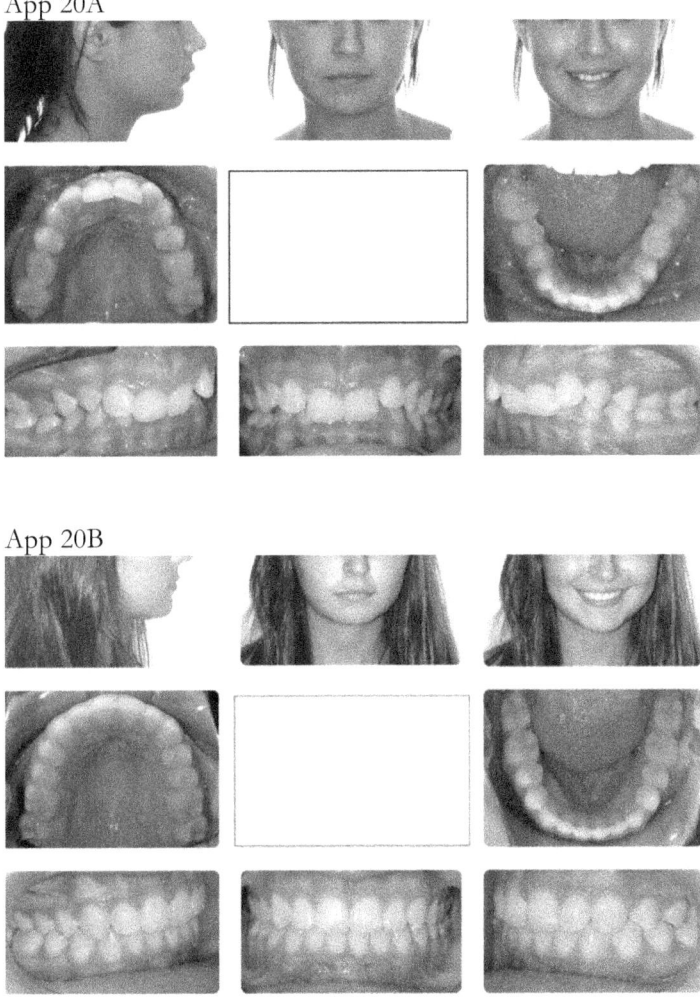

App 20B

App 21A and 21B. Non-extraction treatment. Class II, deep bite, narrow upper arch, and mild crowding. Class II correcting springs were used.

App 21A

App 21B

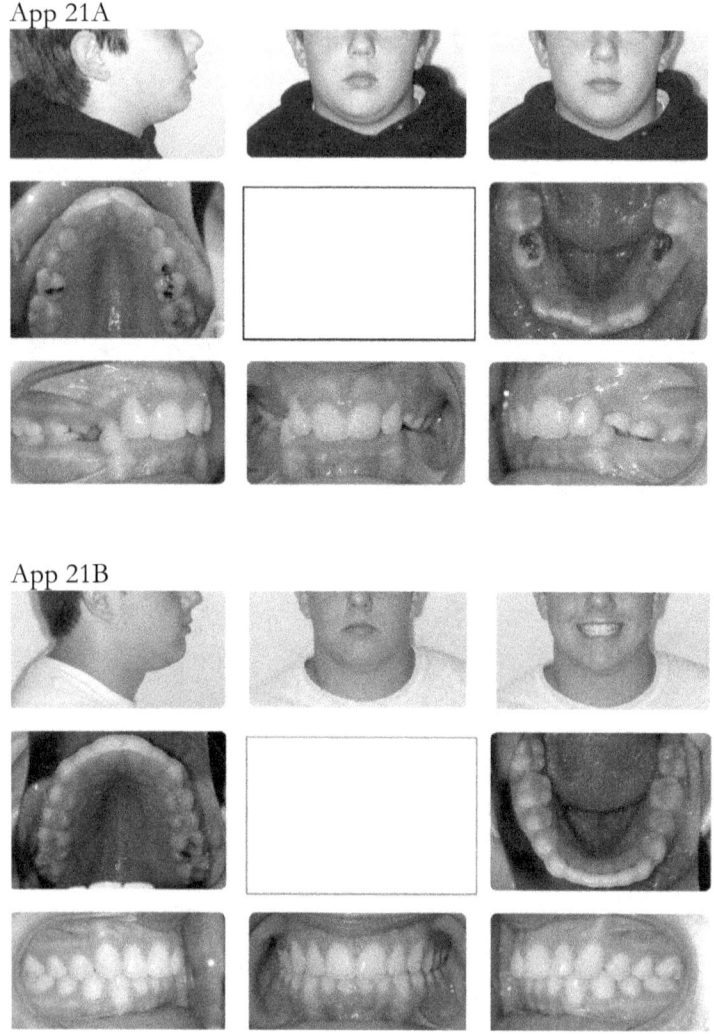

App 22A, 22B, and 22C. Non-extraction treatment. Class I, open bite, thumb-sucking habit, protrusive upper incisors, retroclined lower incisors, and lower crowding. A thumb-sucking habit appliance was worn for about 9 months. The open bite closed and App 22B shows the teeth before the comprehensive treatment started after all permanent teeth erupted.

App 22A

App 22B

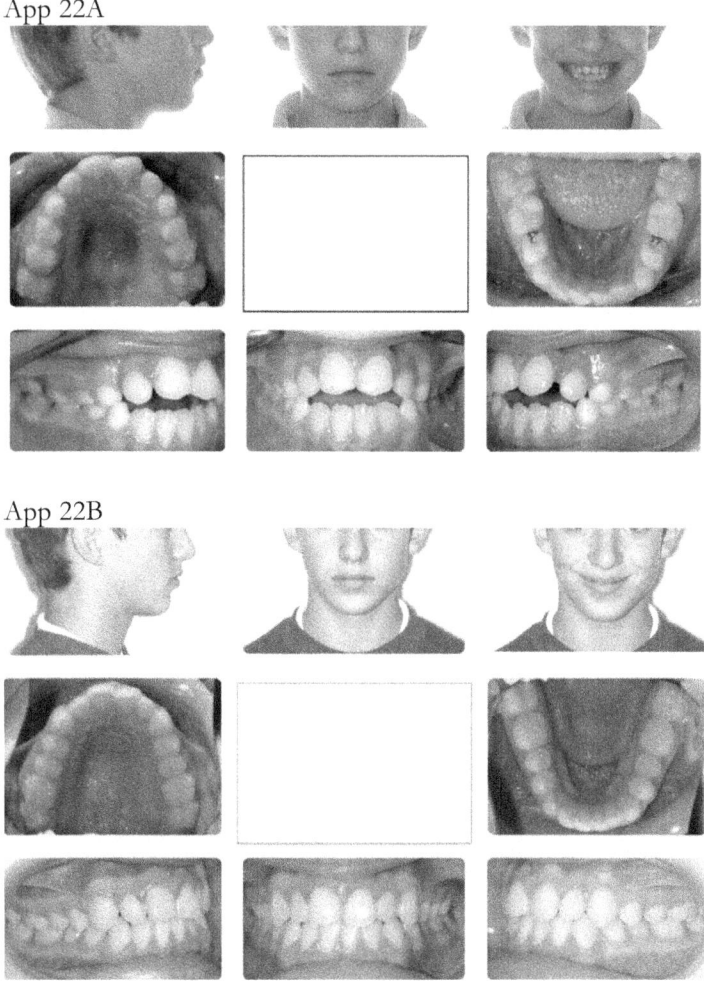

App 22C

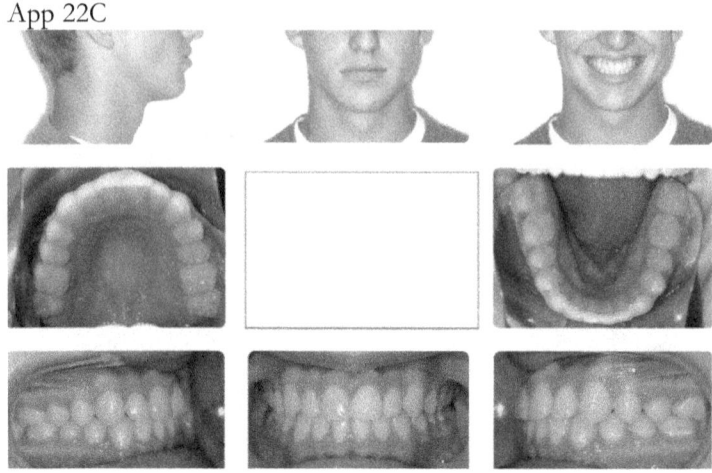

App 23A, 23B, and 23C. Serial extraction treatment and 4 premolars extracted. Class I, moderate crowding, and deep bite. Baby teeth were extracted to guide the crowded permanent teeth. As the permanent teeth erupted, premolars were extracted to make room for the remaining permanent teeth. One comprehensive phase of treatment was completed when all permanent teeth were erupted.

App 23A

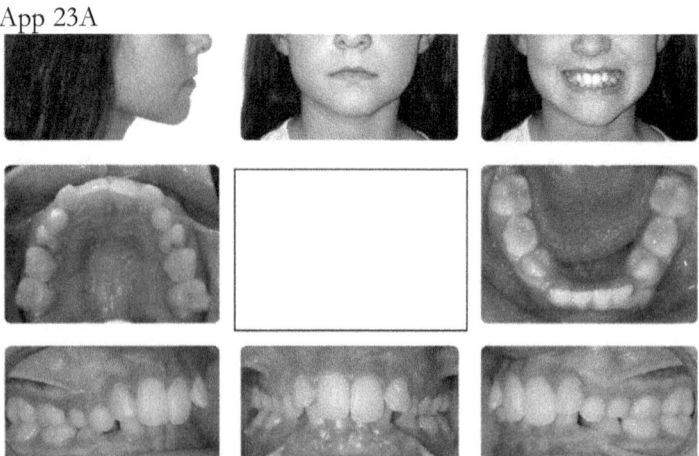

App 23B

App 23C

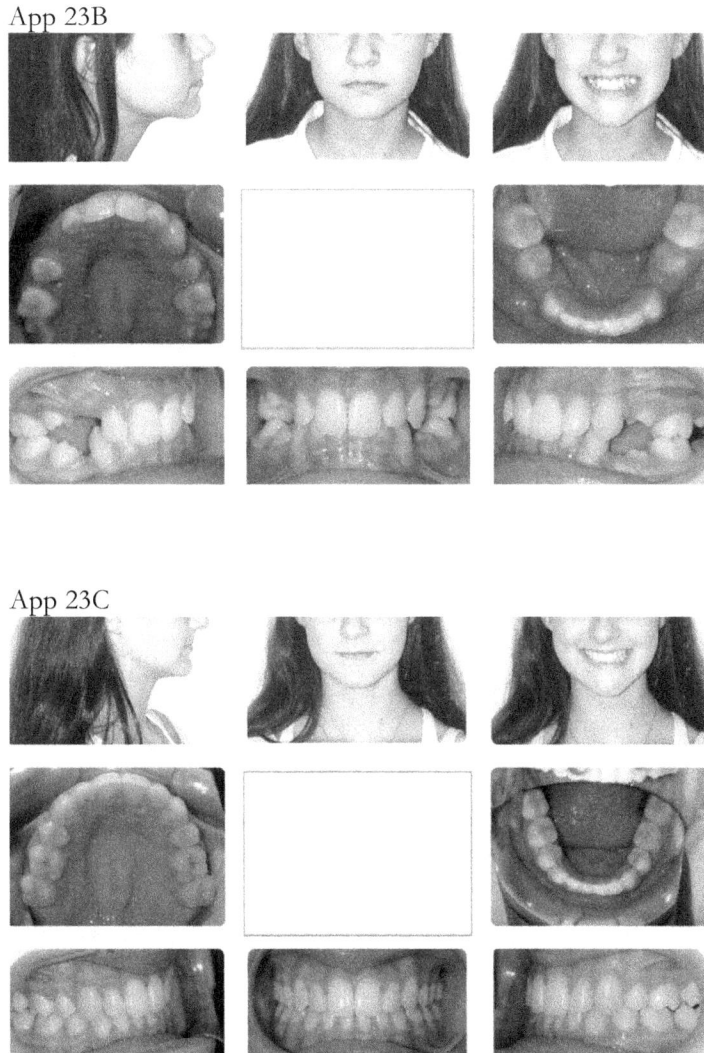

App 24A and 24B. Non-extraction treatment. Class I, large upper midline diastema, and lower crowding.

App 24A

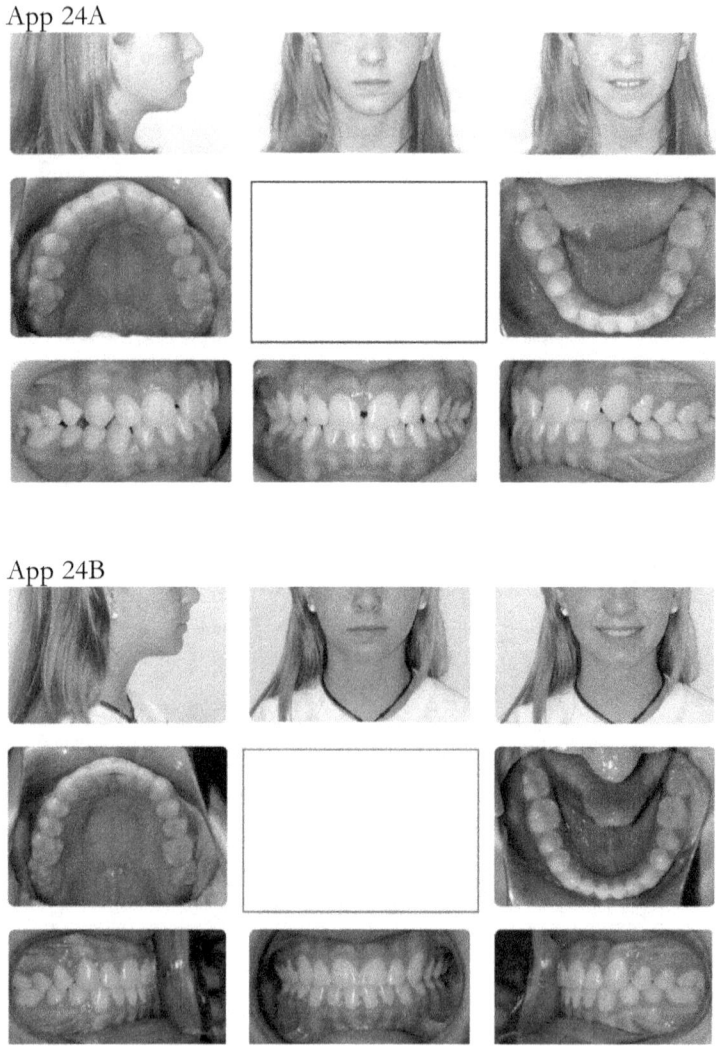

App 24B

App 25A and 25B. Non-extraction treatment.
Class I, upper and lower crowding, and anterior crossbite.

App 25A

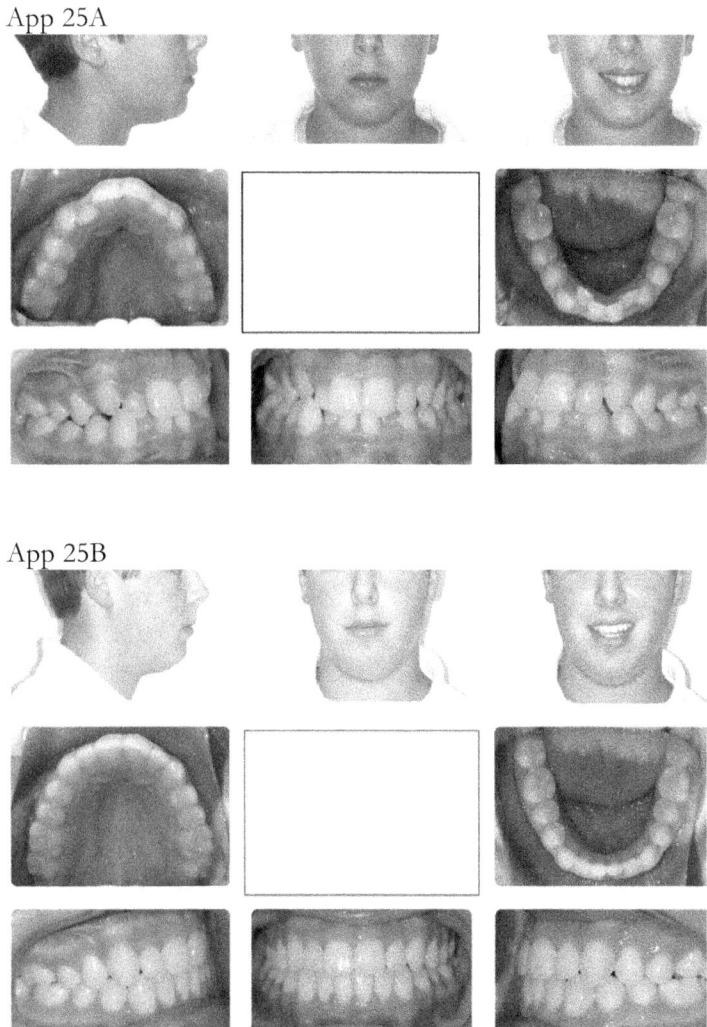

App 25B

App 26A and 26B. Non-extraction treatment.
Class I, upper and lower crowding, deep bite, and narrow
arches.

App 26A

App 26B

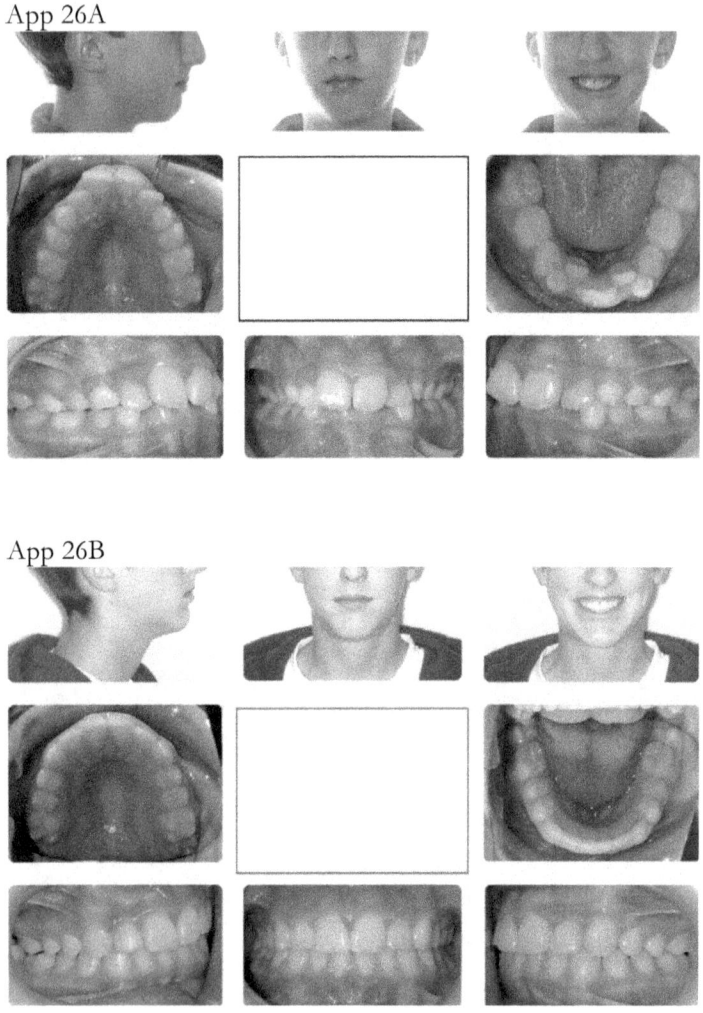

App 27A and 27B. Non-extraction treatment.
Class I, narrow upper arch, posterior crossbite, functional
shift with midline off to the right, and reverse smile line.

App 27A

App 27B

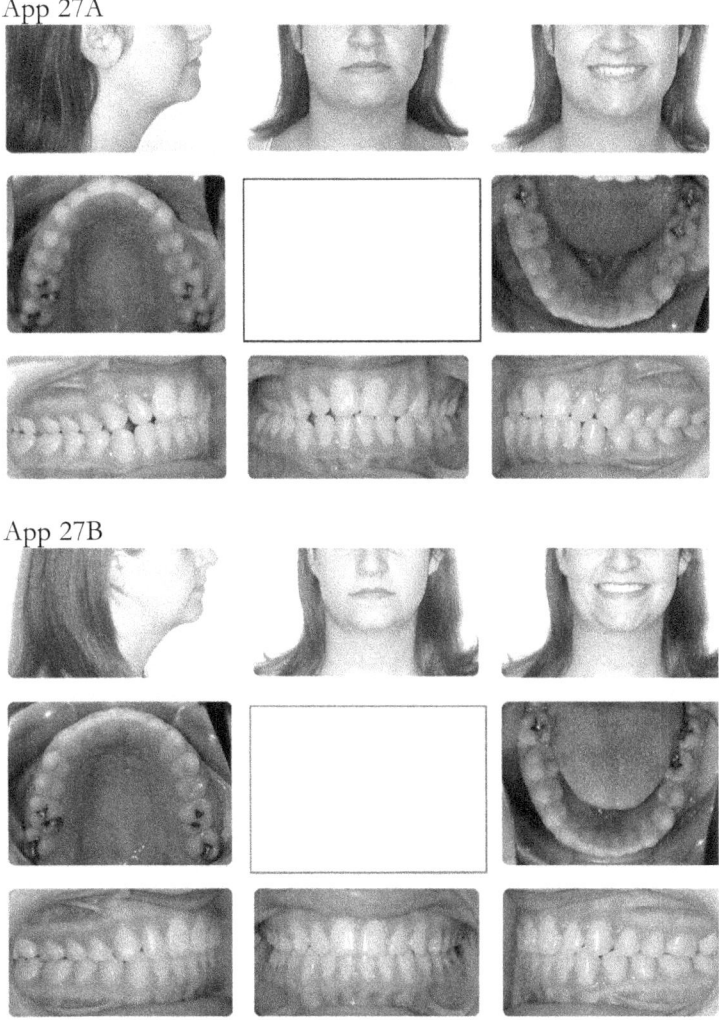

App 28A and 28B. Non-extraction treatment. Class II, upper spacing, protrusive upper incisors, and retrognathic mandible. Class II correcting springs were used.

App 28A

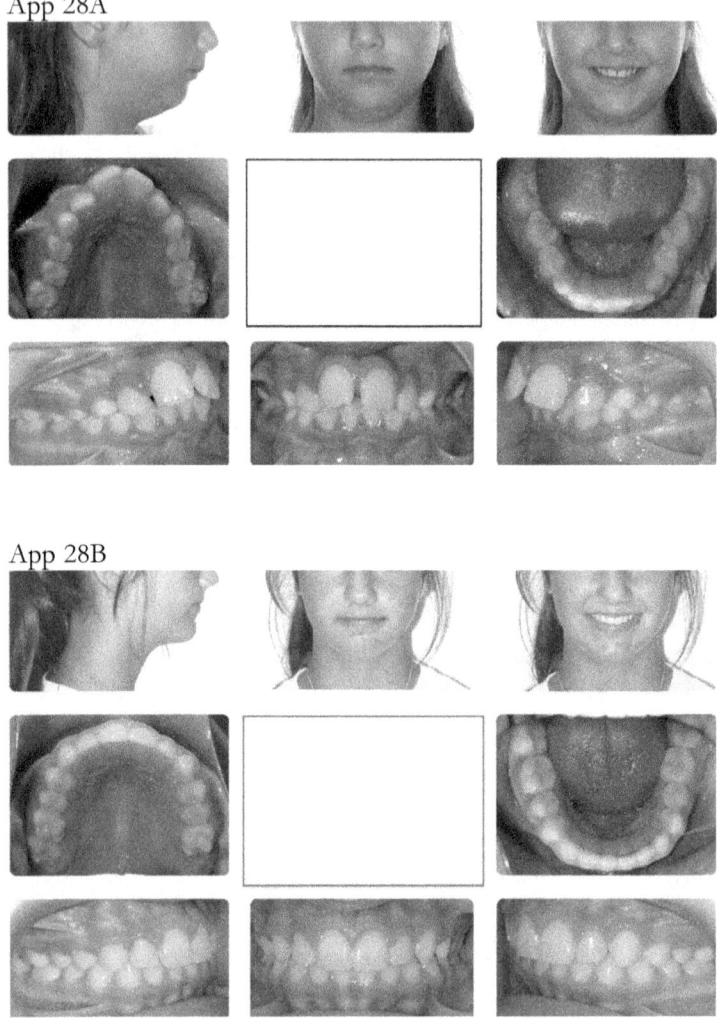

App 28B

App 29A and 29B. Non-extraction treatment. Class I, upper and lower crowding, blocked out and unerupted maxillary right canine, upper midline off to the right, and anterior crossbite. Lower IPR was done.

App 29A

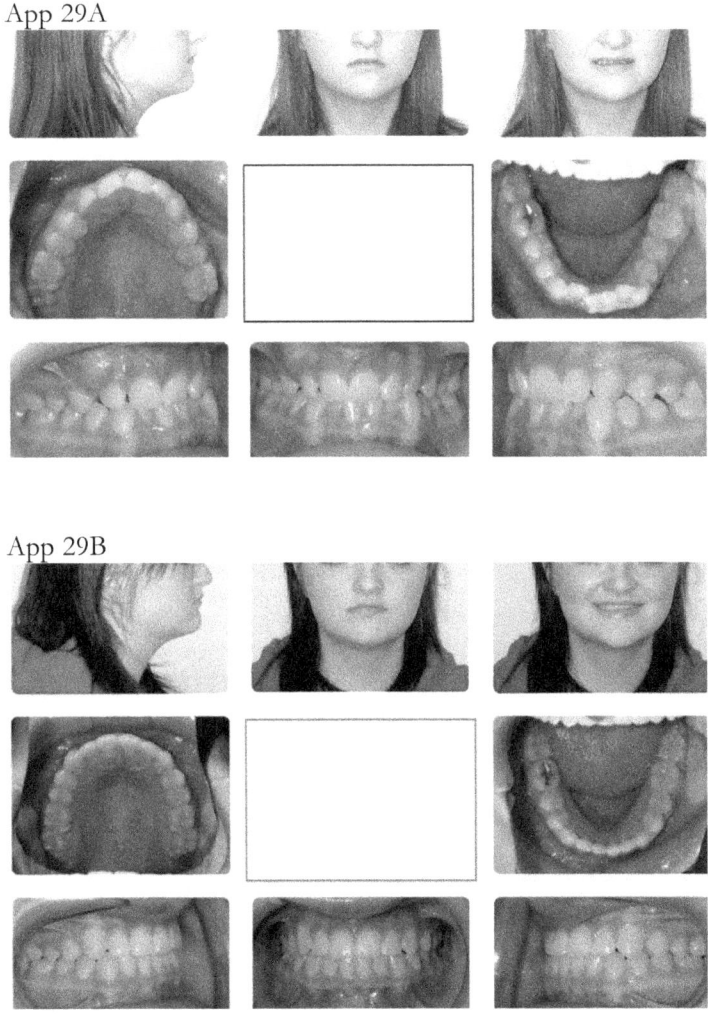

App 29B

App 30A and 30B. Extraction of 2 upper premolars. Class II, upper and lower crowding, protrusive upper incisors, narrow arches, and protrusive lips.

App 30A

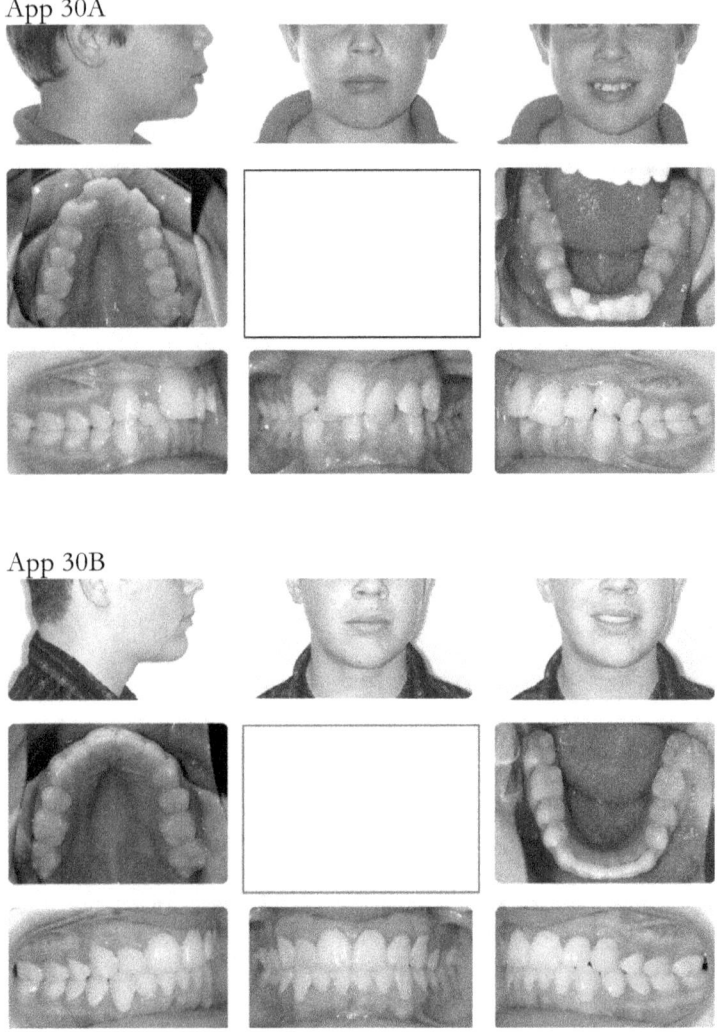

App 30B

App 31A and 31B. Non-extraction treatment.
Class I, midline diastema, upper and lower crowding, and
lateral openbite.

App 31A

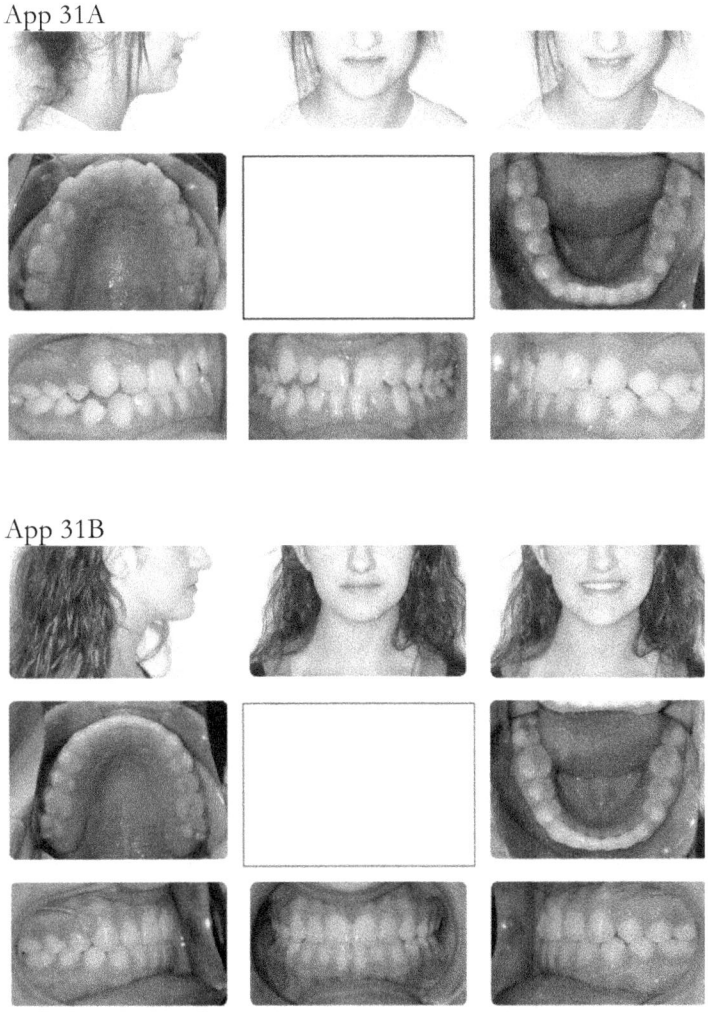

App 31B

App 32A and 32B. Non-extraction treatment. Class I, lower crowding, anterior deep bite, posterior crossbite, narrow upper arch, and lower midline off to the left. A Rapid Maxillary Expander was used.

App 32A

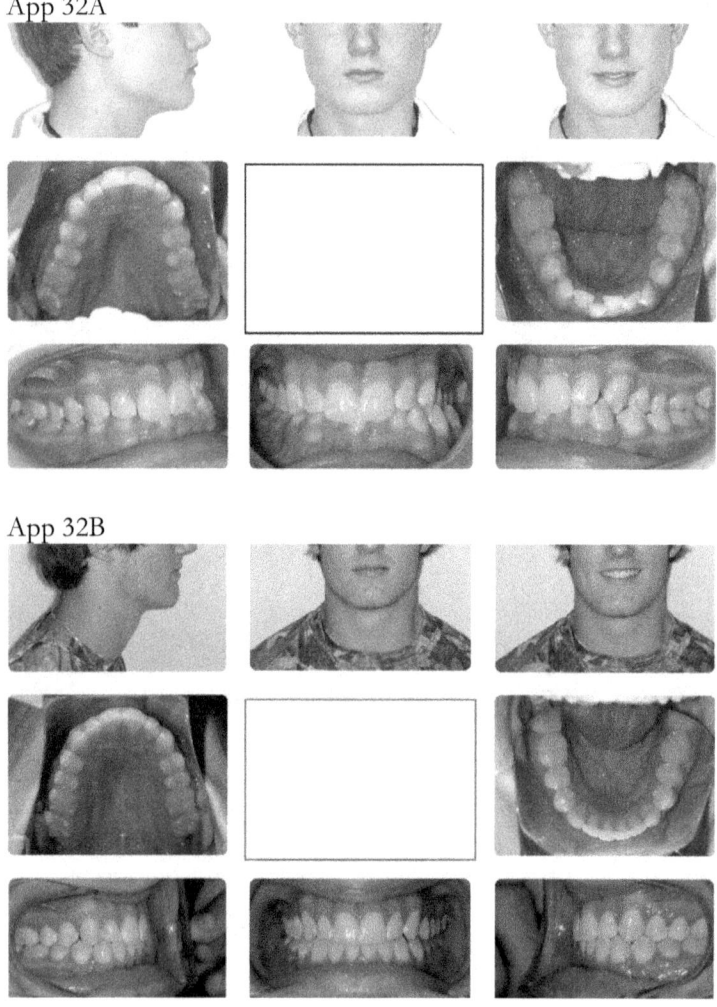

App 32B

Glossary of Terms

3D scan: A form of diagnostic information where x-rays generate more than a two dimensional film of the jaw bones and teeth. On a computer, the orthodontist can visualize and manipulate the teeth and bones of the face and jaws to see the complete structures in three dimensions. These scans can take the place of individual panoramic and cephalometric radiographs.

Anterior: Referring to the front (of your mouth). Anterior teeth include incisors and canines.

Appliance: Anything your orthodontist attaches to your teeth, which moves your teeth or changes the shape of your jaw. A "fixed" or "bonded" appliance remains in the patient's mouth for constant wear; a "removable" appliance is one that is not bonded to the teeth, allowing the patient to take it out his/her mouth for specified periods of time.

Archwire: The metal wire that goes through each of the brackets and allows the teeth to move as if they were on a track. It is changed periodically throughout treatment as your teeth move to their new positions. Adjustments are made by changing the type or size of the wire or by making tiny bends to the wire.

Attrition: Abnormal wearing down of teeth due to function. This results in loss of enamel and tooth structure.

Band: A metal ring that surrounds the tooth and is cemented into place. Bands provide a strong and dependable way to attach brackets/attachments to your teeth or to attach expanders or other appliances. Bands are also a means of attaching a bracket to a tooth with a metal crown, ceramic crown, or filling.

Banding: The process of fitting and cementing orthodontic bands to your teeth.

Board certified orthodontist: An orthodontic specialist who completes the *voluntary* examination process of the American Board of Orthodontics (ABO). Involvement in the certification process is a demonstration of the orthodontist's pursuit of continued proficiency and excellence.

Bond: The seal created by orthodontic adhesives or cements that holds your appliances in place. Brackets are "bonded" and so are permanent retainers.

Bonding: (1) The process of attaching brackets to your teeth using special orthodontic adhesives. (2) The tooth-colored restoration added to small or narrow teeth in order to make them bigger and fill in tiny spaces between neighboring teeth. These are also called build-ups.

Bracket: A metal or ceramic attachment bonded to your tooth that holds your archwire in place. This is another term for the individual braces.

Buccal: Referring to the cheek side of the tooth, closer to the outside of the mouth.

Cephalometric X-ray ("Ceph"): An x-ray of your head, which shows the relative positions and growth of the face, jaws, and teeth. The radiograph is taken of the patient's profile.

Chain (Power Chain): An elastomeric ligature in which the individual O's are linked together to form a continuous chain. This is connected to the braces in order to close small spaces between teeth.

Class I: Orthodontic term used to describe a normal bite.

Class II: Orthodontic term used to describe a malocclusion where the lower teeth fit too far back relative to the top teeth. There is usually a skeletal component to this malocclusion where the mandible is small, and the maxilla is too far forward.

Class III: Orthodontic term used to describe a malocclusion where the lower teeth fit too far forward relative to the top teeth. There is usually a skeletal component to this malocclusion where the lower jaw grew too far in front of the maxilla, or the maxilla didn't grow down and forward enough relative to the mandible.

Coil Spring: A spring that fits between your brackets and over your archwire. It is used to open space between your teeth.

Consultation: A meeting with your orthodontist to discuss a treatment plan, estimated time in treatment, or financial arrangements.

Crossbite: Malocclusion where teeth fit on the wrong side of each other when you bite. Anterior crossbites involve the upper front teeth fitting behind the lower front teeth. Posterior crossbites involve the upper back teeth fitting too far towards the tongue or towards the cheek when they contact the lower teeth.

Debanding: The process of removing cemented orthodontic bands from your teeth.

Debonding: The process of removing bonded orthodontic brackets from your teeth or taking your braces off.

Deep bite: Malocclusion where the upper front teeth vertically overlap too much of the lower front teeth during biting.

Diastema: Dental term for a space between teeth. A midline diastema is a gap between the front teeth.

Direct bonding: The process of placing brackets individually on your teeth.

Elastic (Rubber Band): A small rubber band that is hooked between different parts on your braces to provide pressure in order to move your teeth to their new position.

Elastic Ties, "O" rings, or "O's": The tiny rubber band that fits around your bracket to hold the archwire in place. These are the colors you see on braces, and they need to be changed on a regular basis.

Eruption: The term that describes the movement of the tooth into the mouth. A tooth forms in the gums, and as it "grows" into place and visibly in the mouth, it is erupting.

Facial: Referring to the side of the tooth that faces the cheeks or lips. Braces are most often bonded to this surface of the teeth.

Gingiva: Another term for gum tissue. This is the pink or red soft tissue that surrounds teeth.

Growth modification: Orthodontic therapy used to modify the growth of jaws in children during early treatment. This is part of dentofacial orthopedics.

Headgear: An orthopedic appliance that uses an external wire apparatus known as a facebow to gently guide the growth of your jaws to the proper position. The force is applied to the facebow by a spring-loaded neck strap or head strap. The straps have a safety release that disconnects if the facebow is pulled or snagged. The facebow is attached to bands on posterior teeth.

Headgear Tube: A round, hollow attachment on your molar bands. The inner bow of your headgear fits into it.

Hook: A welded or removable arm to which elastics are attached. Hooks are found on brackets or archwires. They may look like tiny antennae.

Impacted tooth: A tooth that cannot properly erupt to its normal position because of some barrier. Sometimes another tooth can block the path of eruption of a tooth. Other causes of impaction may be thick gum tissue or lack of space. Wisdom teeth are often impacted.

Impressions: The process of making a mold of your teeth by biting into a soft material that hardens into a negative replica of your teeth. Alternatively, digital impressions use a special camera that takes many pictures of your teeth and puts them together to form a digital image of your teeth. Your orthodontist will use these impressions to make models of your teeth and prepare your treatment plan.

Incisors: Teeth found in the front of the mouth. These usually have a single root. There are central incisors (front two teeth) and lateral incisors (next to the front two teeth). These are meant to bite into and cut away pieces of food.

Indirect bonding: The process of bonding brackets to your teeth using a transfer tray. The brackets were previously placed in the tray by a lab technician or the orthodontist. The specific bracket positions the technician or orthodontist specifies in the lab are transferred via the tray to the patient's mouth.

Invisalign®: An alternative to traditional braces, Invisalign straightens your teeth with a series of clear custom-molded aligners. Invisalign can correct some, but not all, orthodontic problems.

Ligation: The process of attaching or tying an archwire to the brackets on your teeth. This can be done with elastic O's, chain, or self-ligating mechanisms built into the bracket.

Ligature: A thin wire that holds your archwire into your bracket.

Lingual: Referring to the tongue side of teeth, closer to the middle of the mouth.

Mandible: The bottom jaw bone.

Maxilla: The top jaw bone.

Midlines (dental): The contact area where the two front teeth touch, or the contact that divides the left and right halves of the dental arch. The maxillary dental midline should ideally coincide with the mandibular dental midline, and middle of your face.

Models: The stone or digital replicas of your teeth that are made using impressions. These are diagnostic pieces of information that are used to study your bite.

Molars: Teeth found in the back of the mouth. These have multiple roots and are larger than front teeth. They are meant to bear most of the forces of eating. There are first molars (erupt at age 6), second molars (erupt at age 12), and third molars (wisdom teeth).

Mouthguard: A device that protects your mouth from injury when you participate in sports or rigorous activities.

Open bite: Malocclusion where there is no overlap or contact of the upper and lower teeth during biting.

Orthodontics: The specialty of dentistry that is focused on the diagnosis, prevention, and treatment of dental malocclusions, which may be a result of irregular tooth alignment (crowding or spacing), disproportionate jaw relationships, or both.

Orthodontist: A dental specialist who completes an orthodontic residency of 2-3 years after completing dental school and specializes in the practice of orthodontics.

Overbite: The vertical (up-down) overlap of your front teeth when you bite. A normal overbite is about 2 millimeters.

Overjet: The horizontal (front to back) overlap of your front teeth when you bite. It is the distance between your maxillary incisors and your mandibular incisors. A normal overjet is about 2 millimeters.

Palatal Expander: A device that makes your upper jaw wider and makes your upper teeth move out towards your cheeks.

Panoramic X-ray: An x-ray that rotates around your head to take pictures of your teeth, jaw, and other facial areas.

Periodontal disease: A problem of the supporting structures of the teeth. The gum tissue and/or bone that surrounds and supports the teeth are compromised. Examples include advanced recession and bone loss around the teeth.

Periodontist: A dental specialist who specializes in diagnosing and treating periodontal problems. Periodontal disease results in gum recession, bleeding gums, and even tooth loss.

Posterior: Referring to the back (of your mouth). Posterior teeth include bicuspids and molars.

Radiograph: A piece of diagnostic information formed with x-ray beams. The orthodontist uses it to study the teeth and jaw bones.

Recession: The condition where gum tissue around a tooth shrinks or disappears. The tooth looks longer, and the root of the tooth may become exposed. This can be the result of traumatic forces to the tooth or brushing too hard. If recession around a tooth advances and sensitivity begins, the orthodontist may refer the patient to see a periodontist.

Retainer: An appliance that is worn after your braces are removed. The retainer attaches to your upper or lower teeth to hold them in place. Some retainers are removable, while others are bonded to the tongue-side of several teeth.

Self-ligation: A feature of some braces that allows the archwire to be attached to the bracket without the need for elastomeric O's or steel ligatures. These braces have a door or clip mechanism that holds the archwire.

Separator or Spacer: A small rubber ring that creates space between your teeth before the bands are fitted. Sometimes a metal separator that acts like a spring is used.

Splint: A specially designed appliance used for TMJ pain. There are a variety of designs that can be made to fit top teeth or bottom teeth.

Temporary Anchorage Device (TAD or Miniscrew): A device that enables the orthodontist to avoid unwanted movements of teeth. It is a screw that is placed in the jaw bone and attaches to the braces.

TMD (Temperomandibular Disorder): A disorder of the TMJ's where pain, popping, clicking, or locking may occur. Comfortable functioning of the jaws is lost, and there may be limited range of motion.

TMJ: The temperomandibular joint. This is the joint where your mandible meets your head. There is a disc that separates the mandible and the skull bones. There is a left and right TMJ. Sometimes pain or headaches associated with this joint are referred to as a TMJ disorder or TMD.

Underbite: Malocclusion where most of the upper front teeth bite behind the lower front teeth. It is usually associated with a Class III bite.

Wax: Wax is used to temporarily stop your braces from irritating your lips. A patient can place a small piece of wax on a rough part of the braces, and this will smooth the surface and alleviate irritation.

Wisdom teeth: Third molars. These are found behind the rest of the teeth in both arches. There may not be enough room for these teeth to come into the mouth. They are likely to be impacted and cause problems such as periodontal damage and inflammation to the teeth in front of them. Wisdom teeth may also cause headaches and pain.

X-ray: A form of electromagnetic energy used to generate an image of bones and teeth on film or on a computer. Sometimes the generated image of the teeth and bone is referred to as an x-ray rather than a radiograph.

About the Author

Dr. J. Luke Chapman is a practicing orthodontist in Louisiana. He is a Diplomate of the American Board of Orthodontics. He has researched and published articles on various topics, including properties of dental biomaterials and the effects of orthodontic appliances on treatment efficiency.

Dr. Chapman married his high school sweetheart, Jennifer. They have two children, Jack and Abigail. He spends much of his time running to catch up with these two busy children. Dr. Chapman enjoys spending time with his family, jogging, playing tennis, creating better ways to treat his patients, and constantly improving his orthodontic practice.

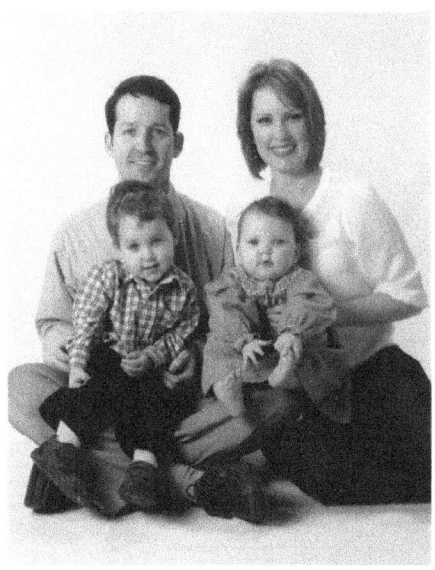

www.ingramcontent.com/pod-product-compliance
Lightning Source LLC
Chambersburg PA
CBHW051702170526
45167CB00002B/507